Workbook for

Sectional Anatomy for Imaging Professionals

Workbook for

Sectional Anatomy for Imaging Professionals

Third Edition

Lorrie L. Kelley, MS, RT(R)(MR)(CT)
Associate Professor, CT/MRI Program Director
Boise State University
Boise, Idaho

Connie M. Petersen, MS, RT(R)(CT)
Adjunct Instructor, Radiologic Sciences Program
Boise State University
Boise, Idaho

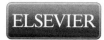

3251 Riverport Lane
St. Louis, Missouri 63043

WORKBOOK FOR SECTIONAL ANATOMY FOR
IMAGING PROFESSIONALS, THIRD EDITION

ISBN: 978-0-323-09419-1

Notices

Knowledge and best practice in this field are constantly changing. As new research and experience broaden our understanding, changes in research methods, professional practices, or medical treatment may become necessary.

Practitioners and researchers must always rely on their own experience and knowledge in evaluating and using any information, methods, compounds, or experiments described herein. In using such information or methods they should be mindful of their own safety and the safety of others, including parties for whom they have a professional responsibility.

With respect to any drug or pharmaceutical products identified, readers are advised to check the most current information provided (i) on procedures featured or (ii) by the manufacturer of each product to be administered, to verify the recommended dose or formula, the method and duration of administration, and contraindications. It is the responsibility of practitioners, relying on their own experience and knowledge of their patients, to make diagnoses, to determine dosages and the best treatment for each individual patient, and to take all appropriate safety precautions.

To the fullest extent of the law, neither the Publisher nor the authors, contributors, or editors, assume any liability for any injury and/or damage to persons or property as a matter of products liability, negligence or otherwise, or from any use or operation of any methods, products, instructions, or ideas contained in the material herein.

ISBN: 978-0-323-09419-1

Content Strategy Director: Jeanne Olson
Associate Content Development Specialist: Amy Whitter
Publishing Services Manager: Hemamalini Rajendrababu
Project Manager: Prasad Subramanian
Designer: Paula Catalano

Printed in United States of America

Last digit is the print number: 9 8 7 6 5 4 3 2

To James,

Min beste venn og evig ledsager,
jeg smiler hver dag på grunn av deg. You are my favorite.
And to Kristina, Matthew, Jennifer, John, Michael, Natalie, Angela,
and Jamers, my greatest treasures, who bless me with their laughter, encourage me
with their unconditional patience and love, and teach me by their selfless examples.
And to my parents, Bill and Darhl Buchanan, for teaching me the value of hard work and for
sharing their wisdom and encouragement in ways that strengthen and inspire me.

LLK

To my amazing husband, Grant, for his constant support and unceasing
faith in me. I love the way I am seen through your eyes.
And to Brady and Trinity, my shining stars who amaze me with their brilliance
every day and remind me of all that is truly important in life.
To my parents, Carl and Ellen Collins, whom I love and admire, thank you for
giving me an endless abundance of strength, love, and encouragement.

CMP

Preface

This workbook is designed to complement the third edition of Sectional Anatomy for Imaging Professionals and is intended to assist and challenge students in reviewing the sectional anatomy and concepts presented in the textbook. It offers a variety of practice items, including anatomy identification, short answer, multiple choice, true/false, matching, fill-in-the-blank, and fill-in-the-table exercises. All chapters in this workbook correspond with those from the text.

The most effective way to use this workbook is to read the chapters in the textbook and then complete the review exercises contained herein.

Lorrie L. Kelley
Connie M. Petersen

Contents

Workbook for

Sectional Anatomy for
Imaging Professionals

Introduction to Sectional Anatomy

OBJECTIVES

1. Define the four anatomic planes.
2. Describe the relative position of specific structures within the body using directional and regional terminology.
3. Identify commonly used external landmarks.
4. Identify the location of commonly used internal landmarks.
5. Describe the dorsal and ventral cavities of the body.
6. List the four abdominal quadrants.
7. List the nine regions of the abdomen.
8. Describe the gray scale used in CT and MR imaging.
9. Describe multiplanar reformation, curved planar reformation, shaded surface display, maximum intensity projection, and volume rendering.

After reading Chapter 1, see if you can complete the following problems.

MATCHING

Directional Terminology

Match each directional term to its correct description.

1. _____ Superior
2. _____ Inferior
3. _____ Anterior/ventral
4. _____ Posterior/dorsal
5. _____ Medial
6. _____ Lateral
7. _____ Proximal
8. _____ Distal
9. _____ Superficial
10. _____ Deep
11. _____ Cranial/cephalic
12. _____ Caudal
13. _____ Rostral

a. On the same side
b. Near the body surface
c. Toward the head
d. Above; at a higher level
e. Toward the front of the body
f. Away from the midsagittal plane
g. The sole of the foot
h. On the opposite side
i. The fleshy part of the hand at the base of the thumb
j. Pertaining to the palm of the hand or flexor surface of wrist or sole of foot
k. Below; at a lower level
l. Toward the back of the body
m. Away from a reference point or source within the body

14. _____ Ipsilateral
15. _____ Contralateral
16. _____ Thenar
17. _____ Volar
18. _____ Palmar
19. _____ Plantar

n. Toward the midsagittal plane
o. Farther into the body and away from the body surface
p. Toward the nose
q. Toward a reference point or source within the body
r. Toward the feet
s. The front or palm of the hand

Regional Terminology

Match the region to its correct location.

1. _____ Abdominal
2. _____ Axillary
3. _____ Calf
4. _____ Cephalic
5. _____ Cubital
6. _____ Gluteal
7. _____ Mammary
8. _____ Pelvic
9. _____ Popliteal
10. _____ Sternal
11. _____ Thoracic
12. _____ Vertebral

a. Back of the knee
b. Head
c. Posterior surface of elbow area of the arm
d. Upper chest or breast
e. Abdomen
f. Lower posterior portion of the leg
g. Spine
h. Sternum
i. Pelvis
j. Buttock
k. Chest
l. Armpit

FILL IN THE TABLE

Fill in the blanks in the following table.
Internal Landmarks

Landmark	Location
	2.5 cm below jugular notch
Aortic bifurcation	L4-L5
	T4-T5, sternal angle
Carotid bifurcation	
Celiac trunk	4 cm above transpyloric plane
	Suprasellar cistern
Common iliac vein bifurcation	
	T12 to L1, L2
Heart: apex	fifth intercostal space, left midclavicular line
Heart: base	Level of second and third costal cartilages behind sternum
	4 cm above bifurcation of abdominal aorta
Portal vein	
	Anterior to L1, inferior to superior mesenteric artery
Superior mesenteric artery	
	Thyroid cartilage
	Midway between superior and inferior border of thyroid cartilage

SHORT ANSWER

1. List and describe the four anatomic planes.

2. State the two main body cavities and describe their divisions.

3. List three organs found in the right upper quadrant (RUQ).

4. List six of the nine regions of the abdomen.

5. Describe what the Hounsfield unit (HU) represents in CT.

6. What do CT numbers greater than zero represent?

7. What does the gray scale represent in MR?

8. Describe maximum intensity projection.

9. Describe volume rendering.

10. List the four planes that divide the abdomen into nine regions.

2 Cranium and Facial Bones

OBJECTIVES

1. Define the three cranial fossae.
2. Identify the location and unique structures of each cranial and facial bone.
3. Identify the structures of the middle and inner ear, and describe their functions.
4. Identify the cranial sutures.
5. Describe the six fontanels within the infant cranium.
6. Describe the structures that comprise the temporomandibular joint.
7. Identify the location of each paranasal sinus and the meatus into which it drains.
8. Identify the structures of the osteomeatal unit.
9. Identify the bones that form the orbit and their associated openings.
10. Describe the structures that comprise the globe of the eye.
11. List the muscles of the eye, and describe their functions and locations.

After reading Chapter 2, see if you can complete the following problems.

MATCHING

Match each cranial bone to its corresponding feature.

1. _____ Parietal   a. Foramen ovale

2. _____ Occipital   b. Carotid canal

3. _____ Frontal   c. Orbital plate

4. _____ Temporal   d. Clivus

5. _____ Sphenoid   e. Cribriform plate

6. _____ Ethmoid   f. Sides of the cranium

TRUE/FALSE

Circle either True or False for each of the following statements.

True/False   1. The largest immovable facial bone is the mandible.

True/False   2. The temporomandibular joint (TMJ) is formed by the condyloid process, the mandible, and the mandibular fossa of the temporal bone.

True/False   3. The maxillary sinuses drain into the inferior nasal meatus.

True/False   4. There is typically only one sphenoid sinus.

True/False   5. The ethmoid bulla is part of the osteomeatal complex.

True/False   6. The inner ear is normally fluid filled.

True/False   7. The vestibule is a structure of the inner ear that controls hearing.

True/False   8. The temporal bone forms part of the bony orbit.

True/False   9. The lacrimal gland is located in the inferior medial portion of the orbit.

True/False   10. A function of the oblique muscle group is to rotate the eyeball.

FILL IN THE BLANKS

Fill in the blank spaces in the following sentences.

1. Located within the basilar turn of the cochlea is the

   _____.

2. The _____ is located at the junction of the brainstem and spinal cord.

3. The basilar portion of the occipital bone is termed

   the _____.

4. The zygomatic process extends from the _____ bone.

5. The _____ bone is shaped like a butterfly and extends across the entire floor of the middle cranial fossa.

6. Located on the lateral surface of the ramus is the

   _____ muscle, which elevates the mandible.

7. The _____ forms the inferior portion of the bony nasal septum.

8. The _____ creates the anterior boundary of the temporomandibular joint, preventing forward displacement of the mandibular condyle.

9. The ethmoid notch of the frontal bone articulates

   with the _____ of the ethmoid bone.

10. The anterior portion of the sella turcica is termed

    the _____.

11. One of the largest of the ethmoid air cells (ethmoid

    sinuses) is the _____.

12. The greater wings of the sphenoid bone contain

    three paired foramina termed the _____,

    _____, and _____.

13. The articular disk of the TMJ is attached to the medial and lateral surface of the mandibular condyle

    by the _____.

FILL IN THE TABLE (see Table 2.3)

Fill in the blanks in the following tables.

Paranasal Sinus Drainage Location

Sinus	Drainage Location
Ethmoid: anterior	Middle nasal meatus
Ethmoid: posterior	
Maxillary	Middle nasal meatus
Sphenoid	
Frontal	

FILL IN THE TABLE (see Table 2.2)

Write in an answer next to the "x" in the following table.

Foramina and Fissures of the Skull

Bone	Foramen/Fissure	Major Structures Using Passageway
Frontal	Supraorbital foramen (or notch)	x _____
	Frontal foramen (or notch)	x _____
x _____	Cribriform plate	Olfactory nerve (I)
Sphenoid	Foramen rotundum	x _____
	Foramen ovale	Mandibular branch of trigeminal nerve (V)
	Foramen spinosum	Middle meningeal artery
	Pterygoid canal	x _____
	x _____	Optic nerve and ophthalmic artery
	Superior orbital fissure	Oculomotor nerve (III), trochlear nerve (IV), ophthalmic branch of trigeminal nerve (V), abducens nerve (VI), ophthalmic vein
With maxillary bone	Inferior orbital fissure	x _____
Occipital	Foramen magnum	x _____
	Hypoglossal canal	Hypoglossal nerve (XII)
Temporal	x _____	Internal carotid artery
	External auditory meatus	Air in canal conducts sound to tympanic membrane
	Internal auditory canal	x _____
	Stylomastoid foramen and facial nerve canal	x _____
With occipital bone	Jugular foramen	Internal jugular vein, glossopharyngeal nerve (IX), vagus nerve (X), and accessory nerve (XI)
With sphenoid and occipital bones	x _____	Fibrocartilage, internal carotid artery as it leaves carotid canal to enter cranium, nerve of pterygoid canal, and a meningeal branch from the ascending pharyngeal artery
Maxillary	x _____	Infraorbital nerve and maxillary branch of trigeminal nerve (V)
Lacrimal with maxilla	Lacrimal groove, nasolacrimal canal	x _____
Mandible	Mental foramen	x _____

SHORT ANSWER

1. Describe the superior orbital fissure.

2. Describe the mastoid antrum.

3. List the structures of the middle ear.

4. List the structures of the inner ear, and describe their function.

5. List the cranial bones that are joined together by the squamous suture.

6. Describe the anterior fontanel.

7. Describe the parts of the hard palate.

8. Describe the anterior and posterior compartments of the globe of the eye and what each compartment contains.

1. On Figure 2.19, sagittal CT reformat of the occipital bone, label the following structures.

   a. _____

   b. _____

   c. _____

   d. _____

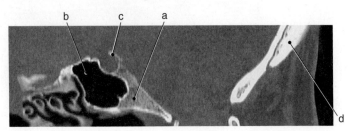

2. On Figure 2.33, axial CT of the temporal bone, label the following structures.

   a. _____

   b. _____

   c. _____

   d. _____

   e. _____

   f. _____

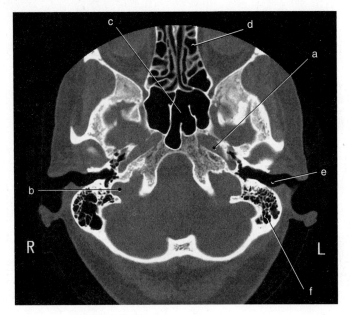

3. On Figure 2.23, axial CT of the sphenoid bone, label the following structures.

a. _____

b. _____

c. _____

d. _____

e. _____

f. _____

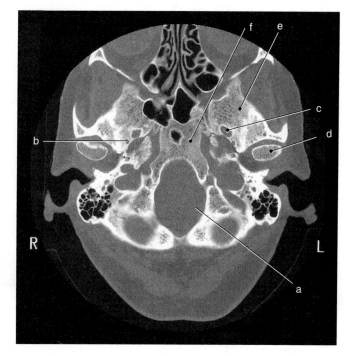

4. On Figure 2.83, coronal CT of the sphenoid bone, label the following structures.

a. _____

b. _____

c. _____

d. _____

e. _____

f. _____

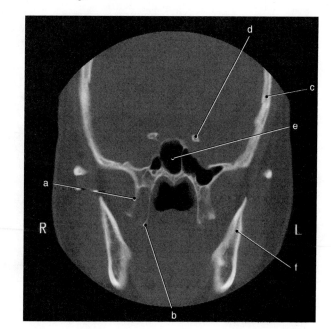

Chapter 2 Cranium and Facial Bones

5. On Figure 2.15, axial CT of ethmoid bone, label the following structures.

a. _____

b. _____

c. _____

d. _____

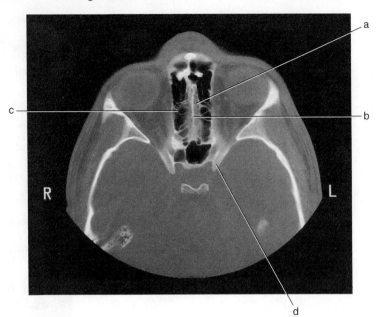

6. On Figure 2.106, coronal CT of the osteomeatal complex, label the following structures.

a. _____

b. _____

c. _____

d. _____

e. _____

f. _____

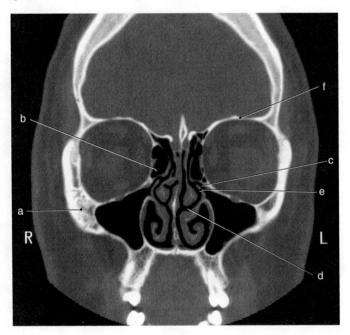

7. On Figure 2.75, axial CT of the hard palate, label the following structures.

a. _____

b. _____

c. _____

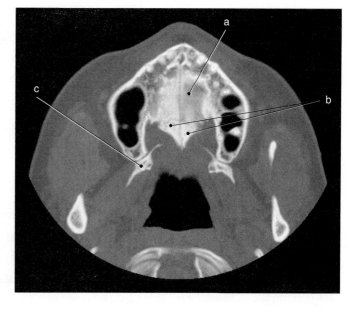

8. On Figure 2.121, sagittal oblique MRI of the orbit, label the following structures.

a. _____

b. _____

c. _____

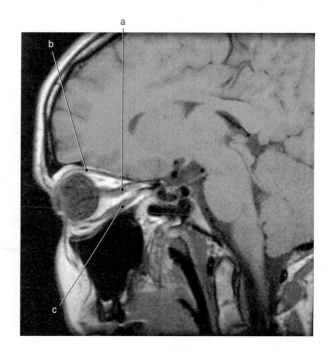

9. On Figure 2.121, axial CT of the orbit at midglobe, label the following structures.

a. _____

b. _____

c. _____

d. _____

e. _____

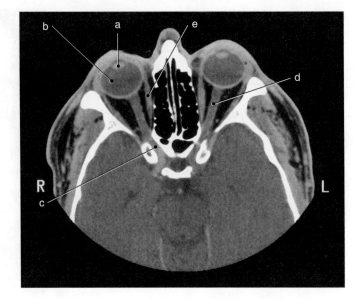

10. On Figure 2.95, axial CT of the temporomandibular joint, label the following structures.

a. _____

b. _____

c. _____

d. _____

e. _____

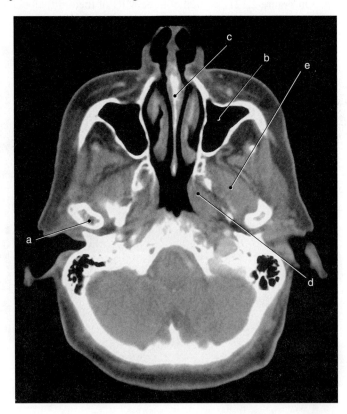

11. On Figure 2.28, coronal CT reformat of cranium, label the following structures.

    a. _____

    b. _____

    c. _____

    d. _____

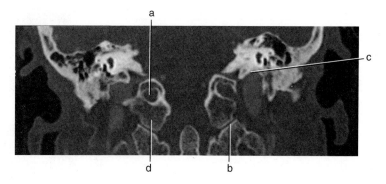

12. On Figure 2.31, sagittal CT reformat of occipital bone, label the following structures.

    a. _____

    b. _____

    c. _____

    d. _____

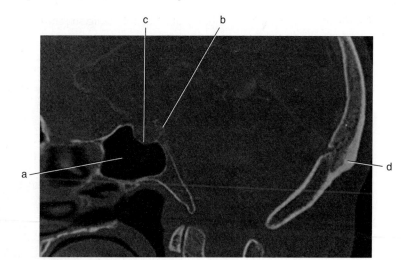

13. On Figure 2.40, axial CT of temporal bone, label the following structures.

a. _____

b. _____

c. _____

d. _____

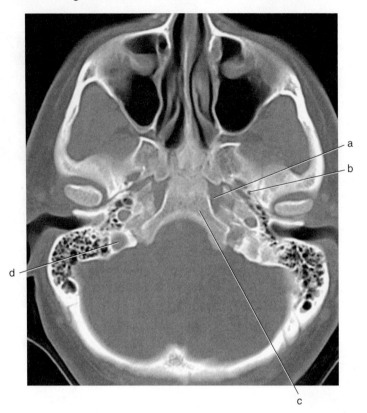

14. On Figure 2.94, axial MRI of head, label the following structures.

a. _____

b. _____

c. _____

d. _____

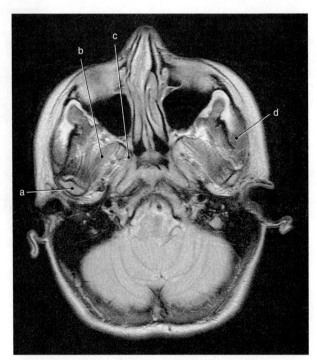

15. On Figure 2.112, coronal CT reformat of cranium, label the following structures.

a. _____

b. _____

c. _____

d. _____

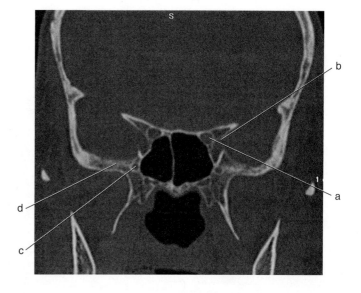

16. On Figure 2.109, 3D CT of bony orbit, label the following structures.

a. _____

b. _____

c. _____

d. _____

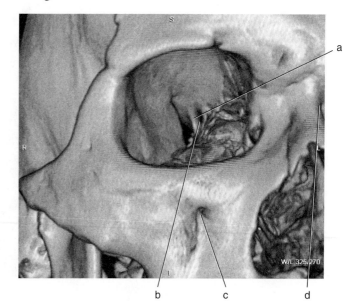

17. On Figure 2.71, 3D CT oblique aspect of facial bones, label the following structures.

a. _____

b. _____

c. _____

d. _____

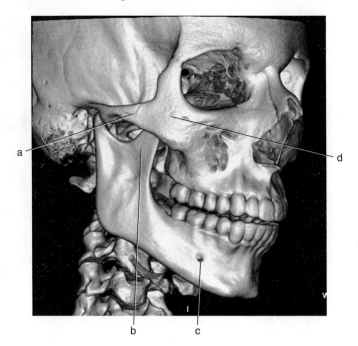

18. On Figure 2.65, 3D CT of 17-week-old infant cranium, label the following structures.

a. _____

b. _____

c. _____

d. _____

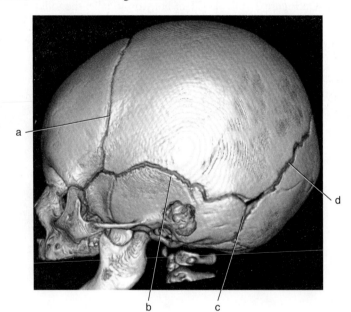

19. On Figure 2.64, 3D CT of infant cranium anterior view, label the following structures.

    a. _____

    b. _____

    c. _____

    d. _____

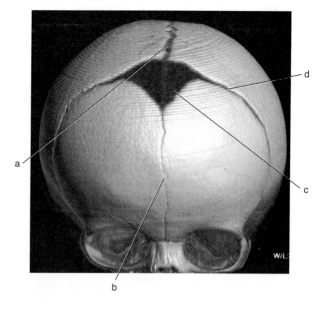

20. On Figure 2.62, axial CT of head, label the following structures.

    a. _____

    b. _____

    c. _____

    d. _____

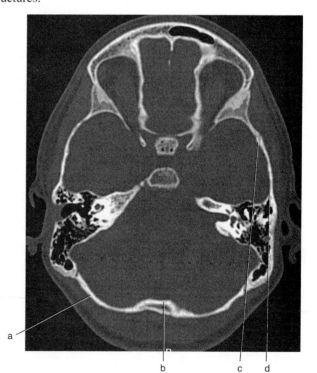

Chapter **2** **Cranium and Facial Bones**

21. On Figure 2.50, CT reformat of middle and inner ear, label the following structures.

a. _____

b. _____

c. _____

d. _____

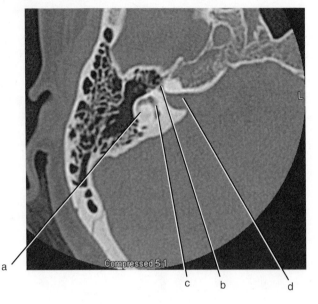

22. On Figure 2.51, axial CT of auditory ossicles, label the following structures.

a. _____

b. _____

c. _____

d. _____

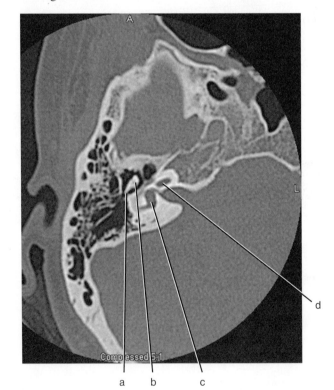

23. On Figure 2.52, axial CT of auditory ossicles, label the following structures.

    a. _____

    b. _____

    c. _____

    d. _____

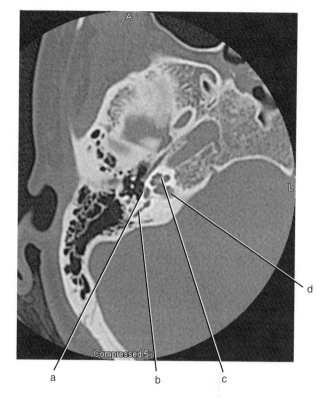

24. On Figure 2.55, coronal CT reformat of middle and inner ear, label the following structures.

    a. _____

    b. _____

    c. _____

    d. _____

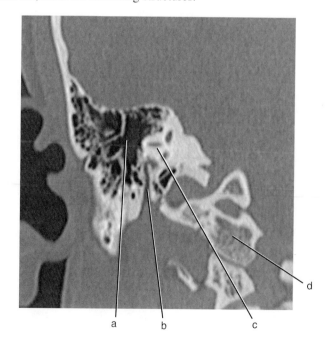

25. On Figure 2.56, coronal CT reformat of middle and inner ear, label the following structures.

a. _____

b. _____

c. _____

d. _____

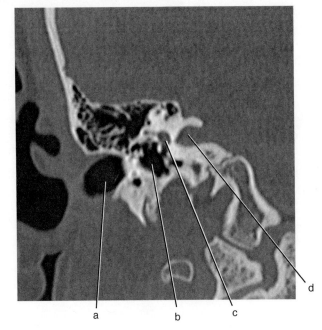

26. On Figure 2.58, coronal CT reformat of EAM, label the following structures.

a. _____

b. _____

c. _____

d. _____

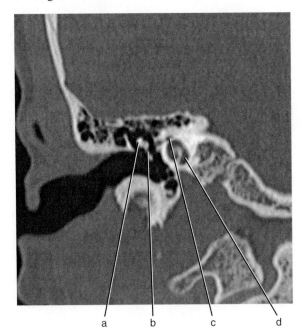

27. On Figure 2.21, coronal CT reformat of cranium, label the following structures.

   a. _____

   b. _____

   c. _____

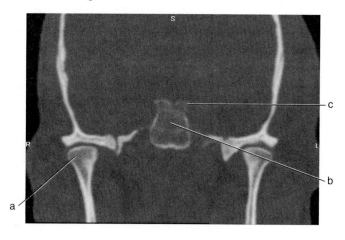

28. On Figure 2.9, 3D CT lateral view of inner skull, label the following structures.

   a. _____

   b. _____

   c. _____

   d. _____

   e. _____

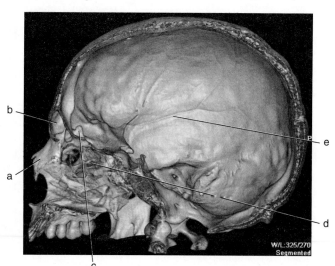

29. On Figure 2.69, 3D CT inferior surface of facial bones, label the following structures.

a. _____

b. _____

c. _____

d. _____

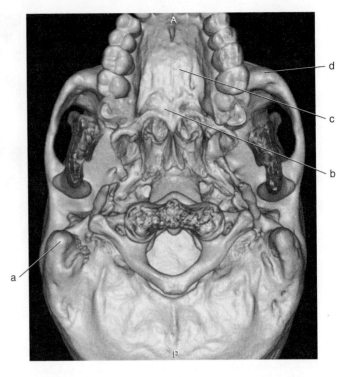

30. On Figure 2.7, 3D CT superior view of cranial fossae, label the following structures.

a. _____

b. _____

c. _____

d. _____

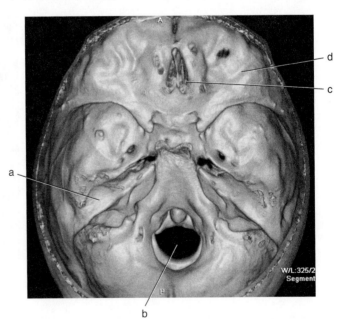

MULTIPLE CHOICE

1. Which cranial bones form the largest portion of the sides of the cranium?
   a. Frontal bone
   b. Parietal bone
   c. Temporal bone
   d. Occipital bone

2. Which cranial bone contains the superior and middle nasal conchae?
   a. Ethmoid bone
   b. Sphenoid bone
   c. Temporal bone
   d. Occipital bone

3. The foramen rotundum is contained in which cranial bone?
   a. Sphenoid bone
   b. Ethmoid bone
   c. Temporal bone
   d. Occipital bone

4. The optic canal is separated from the superior orbital fissure by which of the following?
   a. Greater wing of sphenoid bone
   b. Lesser wing of sphenoid bone
   c. Optic strut
   d. Posterior clinoid process

5. Which cranial bone contains the hypoglossal canal?
   a. Ethmoid bone
   b. Sphenoid bone
   c. Temporal bone
   d. Occipital bone

6. Which of the following foramina is a jagged slit that allows the internal carotid artery to enter the cranium and is located between the apex of the petrous pyramid, body of the sphenoid bone, and basilar portion of the occipital bone?
   a. Stylomastoid foramen
   b. Foramen lacerum
   c. Foramen ovale
   d. Jugular foramen

7. The region surrounding the sphenoparietal suture where the parietal, sphenoid, temporal, and frontal bones meet is termed the:
   a. Pterion
   b. Asterion
   c. Bregma
   d. Lambda

8. The anterior nasal spine is part of which facial bone?
   a. Zygoma
   b. Vomer
   c. Maxillary
   d. Inferior nasal conchae

9. Which part of the mandible contains the alveolar process?
   a. Ramus
   b. Body
   c. Gonion
   d. Mandibular notch

10. Which of the following muscles is the strongest muscle of the jaw, arising from the zygomatic arch and inserting on the ramus and angle of the mandible?
    a. Medial pterygoid
    b. Lateral pterygoid
    c. Masseter
    d. Temporalis

CASE STUDY

Case study 1

A 16-year-old male experienced blunt force trauma to the head. The head CT revealed a basilar skull fracture.

1. Which cranial bones are typically fractured in a basilar skull fracture?

2. Why would otorrhea or rhinorrhea be a possible complication of a basilar skull fracture?

Case study 2

A 9-year-old female experiencing dizziness received a CT examination of the temporal bone that revealed a cholesteatoma of the middle ear.

1. What is a cholesteatoma?

2. As a cholesteatoma enlarges it may destroy the ossicles and adjacent bony structures of the middle ear. What are the names of the ossicles?

3. What are the possible causes of cholesteatomas?

25

3 Brain

OBJECTIVES

1. Describe the meninges.
2. Describe the production and absorption of cerebro-spinal fluid.
3. Identify the components of the ventricular system.
4. Identify the basal cisterns.
5. List the structures of the diencephalon.
6. Describe the location and function of the components of the cerebrum, brainstem, and cerebellum.
7. Identify the structures of the limbic system, and describe their function.
8. Identify the major arteries of the cerebrum, and list the structures they supply.
9. List the arteries that comprise the circle of Willis.
10. Identify the superficial cortical veins, deep veins, and dural sinuses of the cerebrum.
11. Identify the function and course of the cranial nerves.

After reading Chapter 3, see if you can complete the following problems.

MULTIPLE CHOICE

1. Which of the following is not part of the circle of Willis?
   a. Anterior cerebral artery
   b. Middle cerebral artery
   c. Posterior cerebral artery
   d. Posterior communicating artery

2. Cerebrospinal fluid circulates between the:
   a. Dura mater and periosteum
   b. Dura mater and arachnoid
   c. Arachnoid and pia mater
   d. Pia mater and cerebral cortex

3. The dural fold separating the cerebrum from the cerebellum is the:
   a. Medullary velum
   b. Falx cerebri
   c. Tentorium cerebelli
   d. Lamina terminalis

4. Which of the following is not part of the limbic system?
   a. Hippocampus
   b. Mamillary bodies
   c. Olfactory bulbs
   d. Claustrum

5. The white matter tract that connects the two cerebral hemispheres is the:
   a. Anterior commissure
   b. Posterior commissure
   c. Septum pellucidum
   d. Corpus callosum

6. Which of the following does not pass through the superior orbital fissure?
   a. Optic nerve
   b. Trochlear nerve
   c. Abducens nerve
   d. Trigeminal nerve

7. What is the function of the thalamus?
   a. It acts as a relay station for sensory impulses entering the brain
   b. It is concerned with unconscious postural adjustments
   c. It is the primary area responsible for motor control
   d. It contains nerve centers for the regulation of heart rate

8. Which of the following does not course through the cavernous sinus?
   a. Oculomotor nerve
   b. Internal carotid artery
   c. Abducens nerve
   d. Facial nerve

9. Which of the following structures produces cerebrospinal fluid?
   a. Arachnoid villi
   b. Corpus callosum
   c. Ventricles
   d. Choroid plexus

10. The regulation of temperature, appetite, and sleep patterns is a function of the:
    a. Basal ganglia
    b. Cerebellum
    c. Insula
    d. Hypothalamus

11. The fornix connects functional areas of the brain to what structure?
    a. Basal ganglia
    b. Hippocampus
    c. Posterior commissure
    d. Midbrain

12. Which of the following is not a section of the brainstem?
    a. Thalamus
    b. Midbrain
    c. Pons
    d. Medulla

13. What structure separates the thalamus and caudate nucleus from the lentiform nucleus?
    a. Claustrum
    b. Massa intermedia
    c. Internal capsule
    d. External capsule

14. The roof of the midbrain is made up of the:
    a. Tegmentum
    b. Tectum
    c. Lamina terminalis
    d. Pineal gland

15. The cerebral peduncles are part of what structure?
    a. Midbrain
    b. Medulla oblongata
    c. Limbic system
    d. Basal ganglia

16. Which of the following is a linear layer of gray matter lying between the insula and the lentiform nucleus and is thought to be involved with the mediation of visual attention?
    a. Caudate nucleus
    b. Putamen
    c. Claustrum
    d. Internal capsule

17. The walls of the third ventricle are formed by the:
    a. Thalamus
    b. Hypothalamus
    c. Infundibulum
    d. Pituitary gland

18. The midbrain can be divided into which two major segments?
    a. Red nucleus and substantia nigra
    b. Substantia nigra and cerebral peduncles
    c. Cerebral peduncles and tectum
    d. Cerebral peduncles and red nucleus

19. The first branch of the internal carotid artery is the:
    a. Anterior cerebral artery
    b. Ophthalmic artery
    c. Anterior communicating artery
    d. Middle cerebral artery

20. Which of the following dural sinuses begins at the crista galli, runs the entire length of the falx cerebri, and ends at the internal occipital protuberance of the occipital bone?
    a. Straight sinus
    b. Transverse sinus
    c. Inferior sagittal sinus
    d. Superior sagittal sinus

FILL IN THE BLANKS

Fill in the blank spaces in the following sentences.

1. The _____ are located on either side of the anterior median fissure of the medulla oblongata and are described as two bundles of nerve fibers.

2. The _____ is an important structure of the limbic system that has a strong role in transition of memory from short-term to long-term memory.

3. The pontine fibers serve to connect the _____ and the _____.

4. The medulla oblongata contains important vital centers that regulate the control of _____, _____, and _____.

5. The _____ is darkly pigmented and is involved in the production of dopamine in the brain. It functions in the control of muscular reflexes.

6. The function of the cerebellum is to act as a center for _____.

7. The three pairs of nerve tracts that connect the cerebellum to the brainstem are called the _____.

8. The _____ lobe deals with the sensation of smell, taste, and hearing.

9. The _____ fissure separates the frontal and parietal lobes from the temporal lobe.

10. The _____ system is involved in aggressive, submissive, and sexual behavior, in addition to memory, learning, and general emotional responses.

11. The _____ serves to integrate the hippocampus with other functional areas of the brain.

12. The _____ is the middle meningeal membrane.

13. The third ventricle communicates with the fourth ventricle via the _____.

14. The largest and widest bundle of white matter fibers within the cerebrum is the _____.

15. The three portions of the basal nuclei include the _____, _____, and _____.

SHORT ANSWER

1. What are subarachnoid cisterns?

2. Where is cerebrospinal fluid produced, and how is it reabsorbed?

3. Describe the blood-brain barrier (BBB).

4. Which vessels form the circle of Willis?

5. What are the branches of cranial nerve V?

6. Describe the location and general function of Broca's area.

7. List the functions of the frontal lobe.

8. Describe Heschl's gyrus.

9. List the functions of the pineal gland.

10. List four major pairs of arteries that branch from the vertebral and basilar arteries.

FILL IN THE TABLE (see Table 3.5)

Fill in the blanks in the following tables.
Cranial Nerves

Cranial Nerves	Type	Foramen	Function
Optic (II)	Sensory		Vision
Oculomotor (III)	Motor	Superior orbital fissure	
Trochlear (IV)	Motor		Eye movement
Trigeminal (V)	Mixed	Meckel's cave	Multiple
Ophthalmic (V_1)	Sensory	Superior orbital fissure	
Maxillary (V_2)	Sensory		Cheek, upper jaw, maxillary sinuses
Mandibular (V_3)	Mixed	Foramen ovale	
Facial (VII)	Mixed		Facial muscles, anterior two thirds of tongue
Vestibulocochlear (VIII)	Sensory	Internal auditory canal	Hearing, equilibrium
Vagus (X)	Mixed	Jugular foramen	
Hypoglossal (XII)	Motor		Tongue muscles

Internal Carotid Artery Branches (see Table 3.2)

Artery	Region Supplied
Ophthalmic artery	
	Anterior frontal lobe and medial aspect of parietal lobe, head of caudate nucleus, anterior limb of the internal capsule, and anterior globus pallidus
Middle cerebral artery (MCA)	

Vertebral and Basilar Artery Branches (see Table 3.4)

Artery	Region Supplied
	Inferior cerebellum
Anterior inferior cerebellar (AICA)	
	Pons
Superior cerebellar (SCA)	
	Occipital and temporal lobes

1. On Figure 3.70, axial MRI of brain, label the following structures.

a. _____

b. _____

c. _____

d. _____

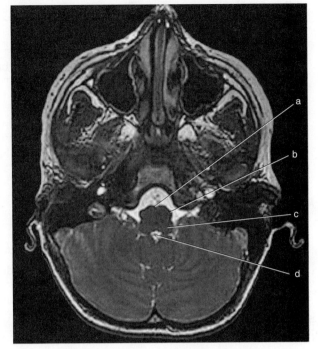

2. On Figure 3.146, axial MRI of brain, label the following structures.

a. _____

b. _____

c. _____

d. _____

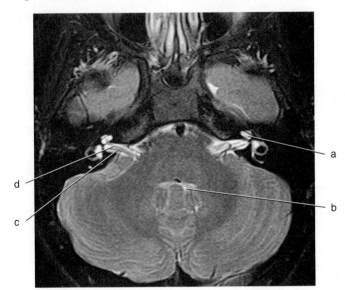

3. On Figure 3.64, axial MRI of the midbrain, label the following structures.

a. _____

b. _____

c. _____

d. _____

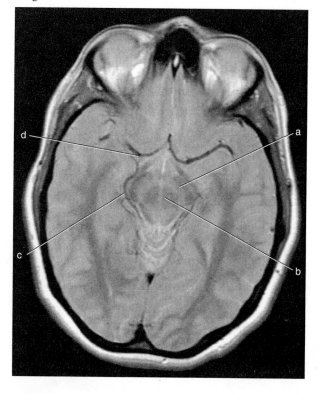

4. On Figure 3.65, axial CT of the cerebral peduncles, label the following structures.

a. _____

b. _____

c. _____

d. _____

e. _____

f. _____

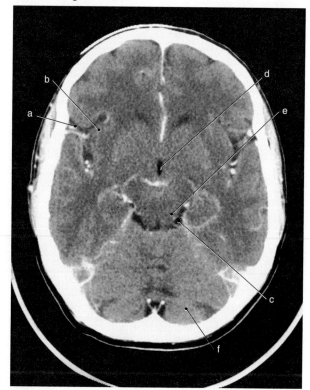

5. On Figure 3.36, axial MRI of cerebral lobes, label the following structures.

a. _____

b. _____

c. _____

d. _____

e. _____

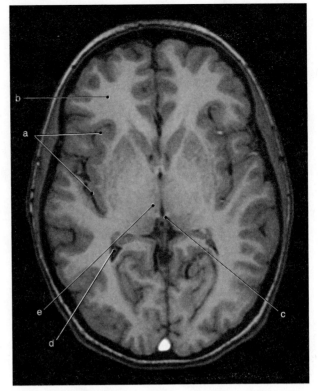

6. On Figure 3.31, axial MRI of brain, label the following structures.

a. _____

b. _____

c. _____

d. _____

e. _____

f. _____

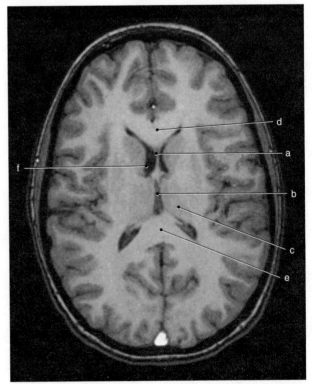

7. On Figure 3.121, axial CT of the brain, label the following structures.

a. _____

b. _____

c. _____

d. _____

e. _____

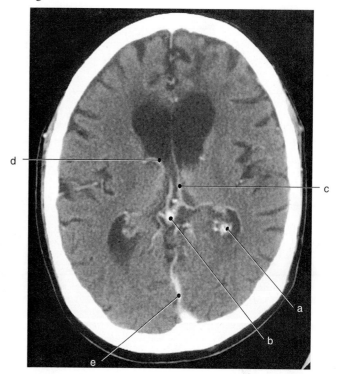

8. On Figure 3.16, coronal MRI of the ventricles, label the following structures.

a. _____

b. _____

c. _____

d. _____

e. _____

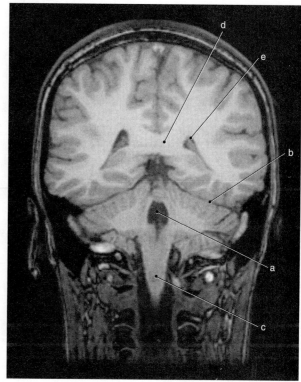

9. On Figure 3.72, coronal MRI of the midbrain, label the following structures.

a. _____

b. _____

c. _____

d. _____

e. _____

f. _____

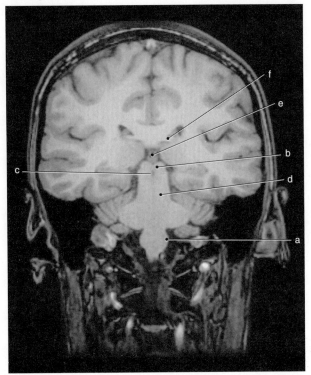

10. On Figure 3.28, coronal MRI of the cerebral lobes, label the following structures.

a. _____

b. _____

c. _____

d. _____

e. _____

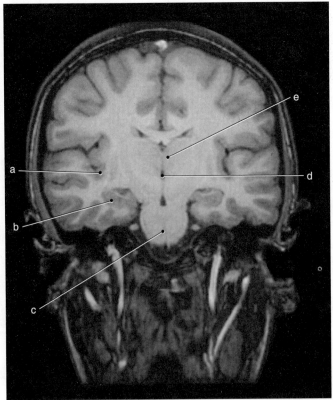

11. On Figure 3.47, coronal MRI of brain, label the following structures.

a. _____

b. _____

c. _____

d. _____

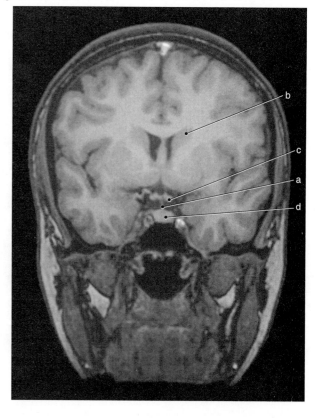

12. On Figure 3.30, midsagittal MRI of brain, label the following structures.

a. _____

b. _____

c. _____

d. _____

e. _____

f. _____

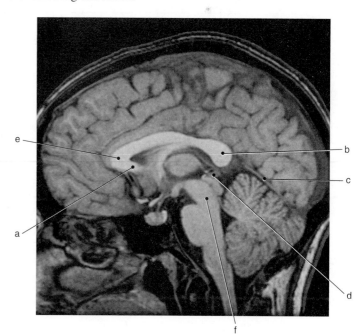

13. On Figure 3.46, midsagittal MRI of brain with corpus callosum, label the following structures.

a. _____

b. _____

c. _____

d. _____

e. _____

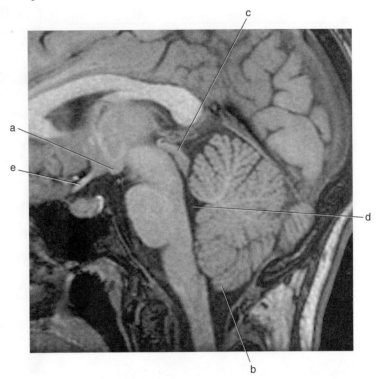

14. On Figure 3.98, coronal CTA of circle of Willis, label the following structures.

a. _____

b. _____

c. _____

d. _____

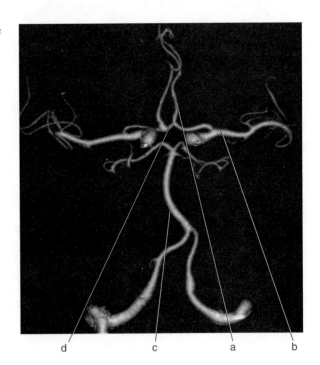

15. On Figure 3.96, CTA of arteries, label the following structures.

a. _____

b. _____

c. _____

d. _____

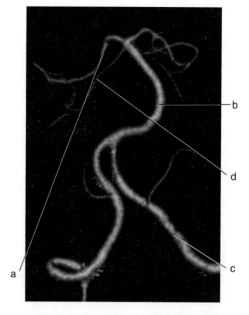

16. On Figure 3.105, sagittal MR venogram (MRV) of cerebral venous system, label the following structures.

a. _____

b. _____

c. _____

d. _____

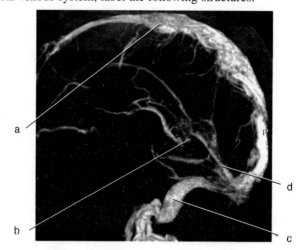

17. On Figure 3.15, coronal MRI of brain, label the following structures.

a. _____

b. _____

c. _____

d. _____

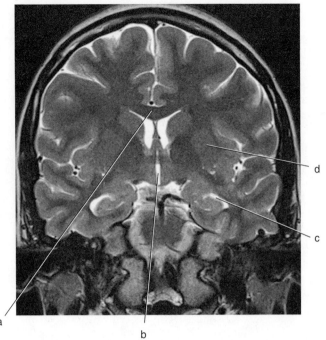

18. On Figure 3.87, submentovertex CTA, label the following structures.

a. _____

b. _____

c. _____

d. _____

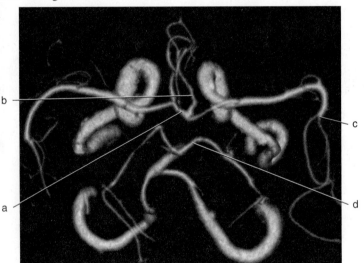

19. On Figure 3.10, axial MRI of brain, label the following structures.

a. _____

b. _____

c. _____

d. _____

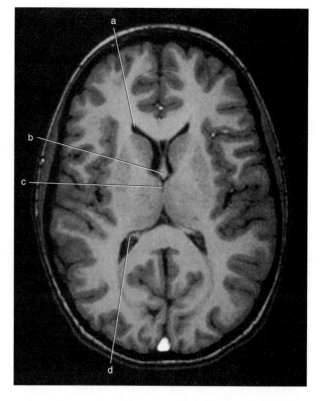

20. On Figure 3.12, axial CT of brain, label the following structures.

a. _____

b. _____

c. _____

d. _____

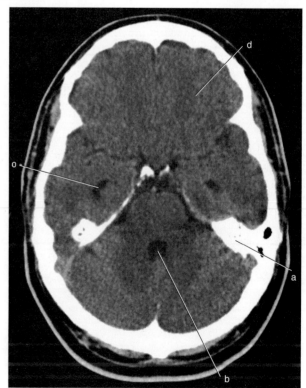

21. On Figure 3.21, axial MRI of brain, label the following structures.

a. _____

b. _____

c. _____

d. _____

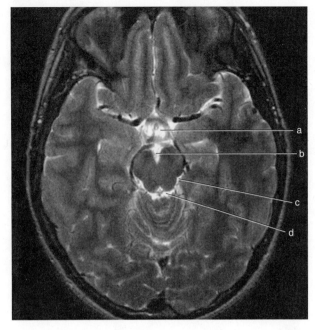

22. On Figure 3.34, axial MRI of brain, label the following structures.

a. _____

b. _____

c. _____

d. _____

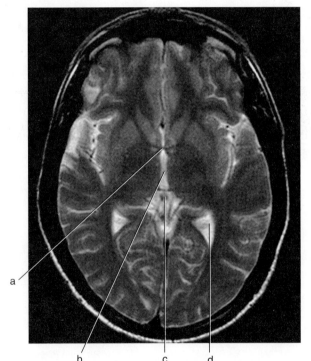

23. On Figure 3.44, coronal MRI of brain, label the following structures.

a. _____

b. _____

c. _____

d. _____

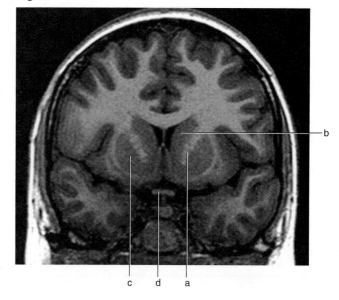

24. On Figure 3.48, coronal CT reformat of brain, label the following structures.

a. _____

b. _____

c. _____

d. _____

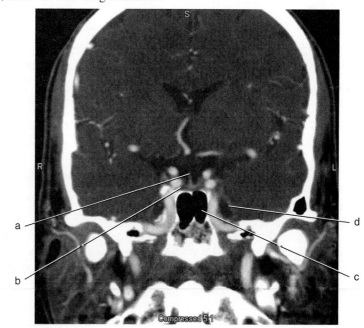

25. On Figure 3.57, coronal MRI of brain, label the following structures.

a. _____

b. _____

c. _____

d. _____

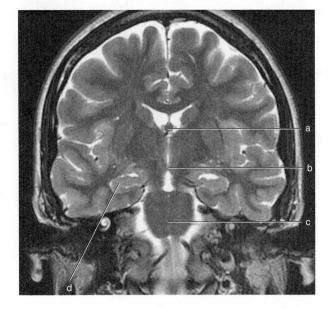

26. On Figure 3.83, axial CT of cranium, label the following structures.

a. _____

b. _____

c. _____

d. _____

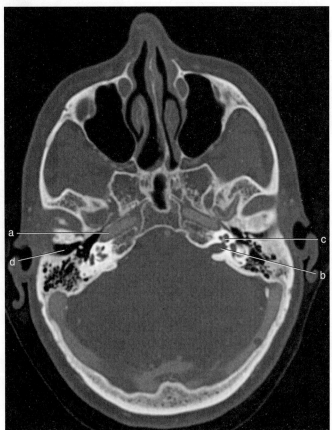

27. On Figure 3.86, sagittal MRA of cerebral arteries, label the following structures.

a. _____

b. _____

c. _____

d. _____

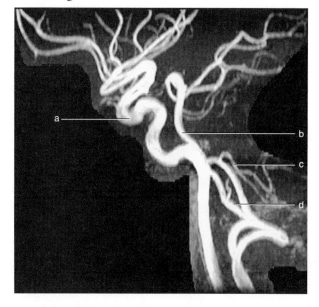

28. On Figure 3.100, axial MRA of circle of Willis, label the following structures.

a. _____

b. _____

c. _____

d. _____

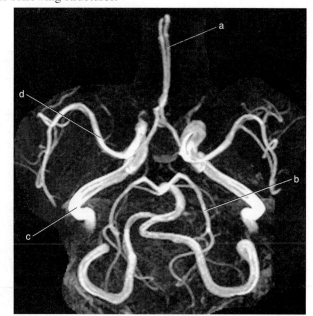

29. On Figure 3.126, midsagittal MRI of brain, label the following structures.

a. _____

b. _____

c. _____

d. _____

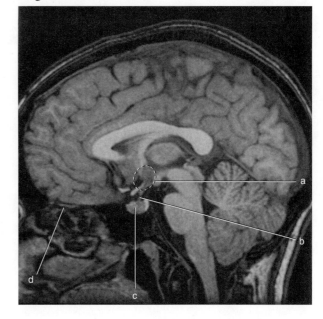

30. On Figure 3.19, coronal CT reformat of brain, label the following structures.

a. _____

b. _____

c. _____

d. _____

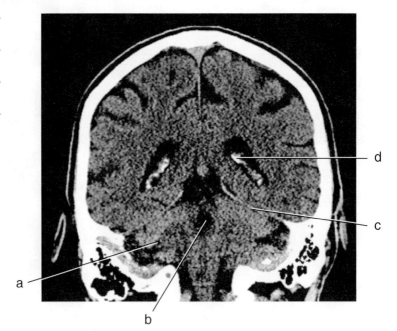

31. On Figure 3.23, axial, MRI of brain, label the following structures.

a. _____

b. _____

c. _____

d. _____

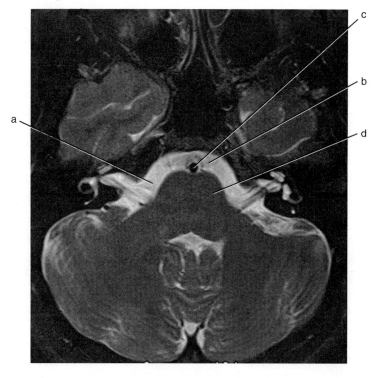

32. On Figure 3.37, coronal CT reformat of cerebral lobes, label the following structures.

a. _____

b. _____

c. _____

d. _____

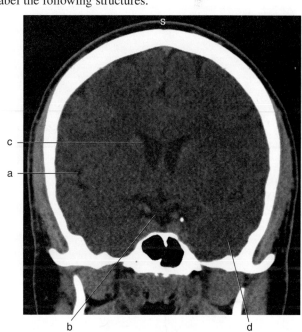

47

33. On Figure 3.69, sagittal CT reformat of pons, label the following structures.

a. _____

b. _____

c. _____

d. _____

e. _____

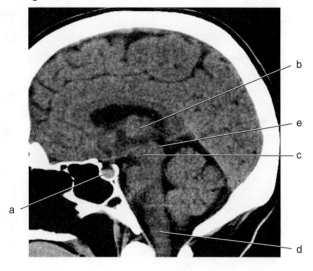

34. On Figure 3.85, lateral CTA of cerebral arteries, label the following structures.

a. _____

b. _____

c. _____

d. _____

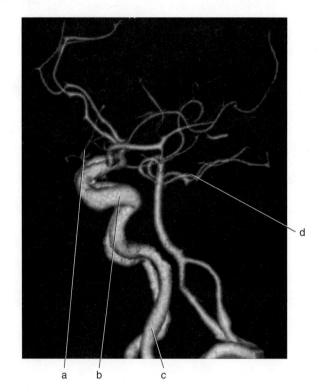

35. On Figure 3.90, axial CT of brain, label the following structures.

a. _____

b. _____

c. _____

d. _____

e. _____

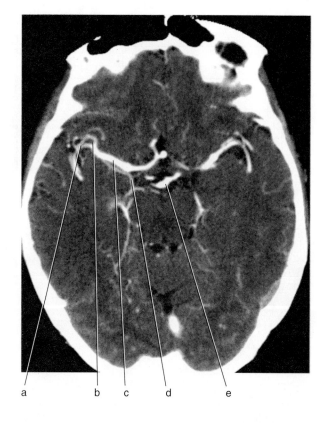

36. On Figure 3.116, coronal MRI of cavernous sinus with contrast enhancement, label the following structures.

a. _____

b. _____

c. _____

d. _____

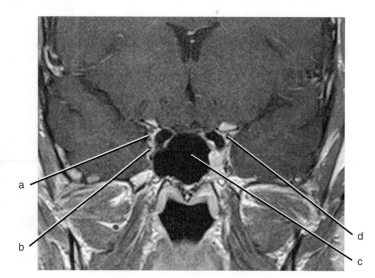

37. On Figure 3.56, coronal MRI of brain, label the following structures.

a. _____

b. _____

c. _____

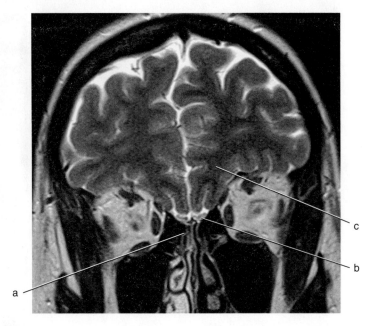

38. On Figure 3.135, axial MRI of brain, label the following structures.

a. _____

b. _____

c. _____

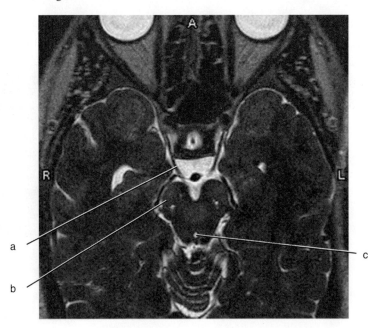

39. On Figure 3.136, axial MRI of brain, label the following structures.

a. _____

b. _____

c. _____

d. _____

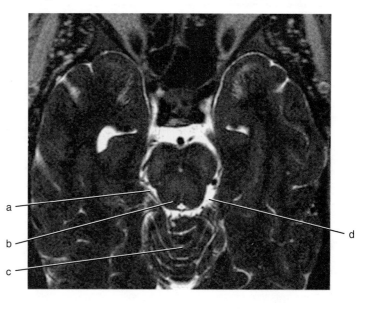

40. On Figure 3.150, axial MRI of brain, label the following structures.

a. _____

b. _____

c. _____

d. _____

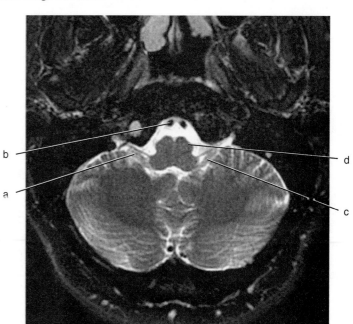

CASE STUDIES

Case Study 1

Skull fractures with rupture of the meningeal arteries can cause a life-threatening condition known as an epidural hematoma (EDH) which causes an accumulation of blood in the epidural space. A subdural hematoma (SDH) is a collection of blood from ruptured vessels located in the subdural space.

1. Where is the epidural space located?

2. Describe the subdural space.

Case Study 2

A patient presented to the emergency department with a severe headache. The head CT revealed a subarachnoid hemorrhage (SAH).

1. What is the most common cause of a SAH?

2. Where would blood collect due to a SAH?

Case Study 3

A patient is scheduled for an MRI of the head to evaluate an AVM.

1. What is an AVM?

2. What are the symptoms of an AVM?

3. How frequently do AVMs rupture?

4 Spine

OBJECTIVES

1. Identify the structures of a typical vertebra.
2. Identify the atypical structures of the atlas and axis, thoracic vertebrae, sacrum, and coccyx.
3. Identify and state the function of the spinal ligaments.
4. Define the action of and identify the muscle groups of the spine.
5. Describe the components of the spinal cord and spinal nerves.
6. List the four plexuses of the spinal cord, and describe the structures they innervate.
7. Identify the vasculature of the spine and spinal cord.

After reading Chapter 4, see if you can complete the following problems.

MULTIPLE CHOICE

1. Which of the following spinal ligaments extends across the vertebral foramen of C1 to form a sling over the posterior surface of the odontoid process?
   a. Alar ligament
   b. Supraspinous ligament
   c. Anterior longitudinal ligament
   d. Transverse ligament

2. An expansive ligament that extends from the external occipital protuberance of the cranium to the spinous processes of the cervical vertebrae is the:
   a. Ligamentum nuchae
   b. Supraspinous ligament
   c. Transverse ligament
   d. Apical ligament

3. Which of the following ligaments is a continuation of the ligamentum nuchae?
   a. Anterior longitudinal ligament
   b. Posterior longitudinal ligament
   c. Supraspinous ligament
   d. Apical ligament

4. Massive muscles that form a prominent bulge on each side of the vertebral column are the:
   a. Erector spinae muscles
   b. Splenius muscles
   c. Transversospinal muscles
   d. Semispinalis muscles

5. Which of the following deep muscles consisting of many fibrous bundles that extend the full length of the spine are the most prominent in the lumbar region?
   a. Semispinalis muscles
   b. Multifidus muscles
   c. Splenius muscles
   d. Erector spinae muscles

6. A potential space called the subdural space runs between the:
   a. Arachnoid mater and the pia mater
   b. Arachnoid mater and dura mater
   c. Dura mater and pia mater
   d. Pia mater and spinal cord

7. The dura mater extends to approximately which vertebral level?
   a. L3
   b. L5
   c. S2
   d. S4

8. Which of the following contain the nerve cell bodies of the efferent (motor) neurons?
   a. Dorsal roots
   b. Dorsal horns
   c. Ventral roots
   d. Ventral horns

9. The largest branch of the lumbar plexus descending beneath the inguinal ligament is the:
   a. Phrenic nerve
   b. Femoral nerve
   c. Sciatic nerve
   d. Tibial nerve

10. Which of the following arteries is formed just caudal to the basilar artery, by the union of two small branches of the vertebral arteries?
    a. Anterior spinal artery
    b. Posterior spinal artery
    c. Anterior radicular artery
    d. Posterior radicular artery

FILL IN THE BLANKS

1. The _____ are extensions of the pia mater; they attach to the dura mater to prevent movement of the spinal cord within the spinal canal.

2. The two _____ project from the vertebral body to meet with two laminae that continue posterior and medial to form a _____ process.

3. The _____ plexus arises from the ventral rami of C5-C8 and T1.

4. The ventral horns contain the nerve cell bodies of the _____ neurons.

5. The conus medullaris is located at approximately the level of _____.

6. _____ veins drain the bodies of the vertebra before joining the anterior and internal venous plexuses.

7. The _____ nerve is the largest nerve in the body.

8. The _____ muscles are superficial bandagelike muscles that originate on the spinous processes of C7-T6 and the inferior half of the ligamentum nuchae.

9. The _____ of the cervical vertebrae allow for the passage of vertebral arteries and veins as they ascend to and descend from the head.

10. There are _____ pairs of spinal nerves that exit the spinal cord.

SHORT ANSWER

1. State the two components that make up the intervertebral disk.

2. Which muscle group is considered the chief extensor of the vertebral column?

3. Which ligaments join the laminae of adjacent vertebral arches to help preserve the normal curvature of the spine?

4. List the structures that make up the vertebral arch.

5. Describe the costal facets of the thoracic vertebrae.

6. Describe the configuration of the white and gray matter within the spinal cord.

7. Describe the cervical plexus, and list its major motor branch.

8. The sciatic nerve descends vertically along the posterior thigh to divide into which nerves?

9. Describe the venous plexuses of the vertebral column.

10. List the three vertical columns of the erector spinae muscle groups.

TRUE/FALSE

Circle either True or False for each of the following statements.

True/False 1. C7 does not typically have a bifid spinous process.

True/False 2. The denticulate ligaments are extensions of the pia mater in the spine.

True/False 3. The deepest spinal muscle group is the erector spinae group.

True/False 4. The filum terminale anchors the spinal cord to the coccyx.

True/False 5. The cervical plexus arises from the ventral rami of C2-C7.

True/False 6. The alar ligaments are two strong bands that extend from the sides of the odontoid process to the lateral margins of the occipital condyles to limit rotation and flexion of the head.

True/False 7. The apical ligament is sometimes called the cruciform ligament because of its crosslike appearance.

True/False 8. The anterior longitudinal ligament extends downward from C1 along the entire length of the anterior surface of the vertebral bodies to the sacrum.

True/False 9. The arachnoid mater is a thin transparent membrane that is attached to the inner surface of the dura mater.

True/False 10. The central canal of the spinal cord contains cerebrospinal fluid but is not continuous with the ventricles of the brain.

1. On Figure 4.10, axial CT of the lumbar spine with intervertebral disk, label the following structures.

a. _____

b. _____

c. _____

d. _____

e. _____

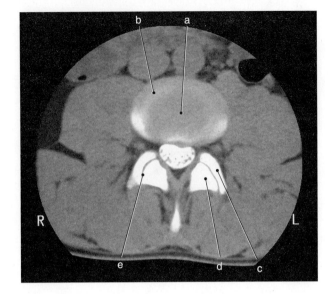

2. On Figure 4.4, axial CT of the lumbar vertebra, label the following structures.

a. _____

b. _____

c. _____

d. _____

e. _____

f. _____

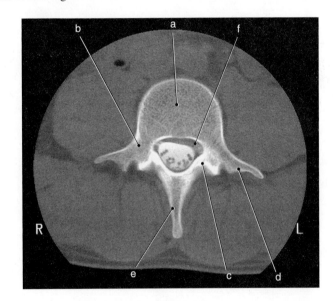

3. On Figure 4.71, midsagittal MRI of the lumbar spine, label the following structures.

a. _____

b. _____

c. _____

d. _____

e. _____

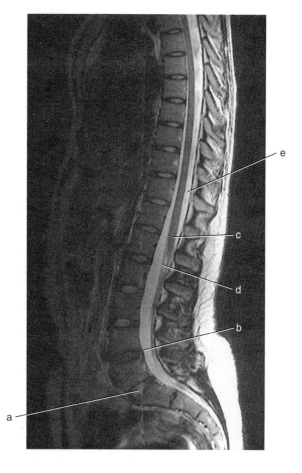

4. On Figure 4.14, axial CT of C1, label the following structures.

a. _____

b. _____

c. _____

d. _____

e. _____

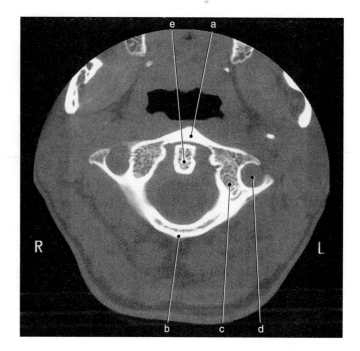

5. On Figure 4.37, coronal CT of the sacrum, label the following structures.

a. _____

b. _____

c. _____

d. _____

e. _____

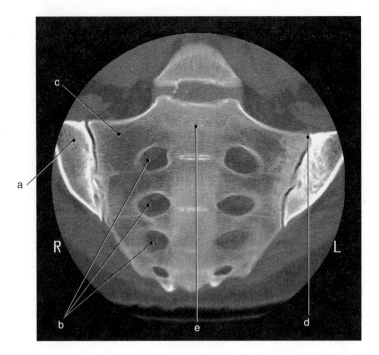

6. On Figure 4.45, axial MRI of the cervical vertebra, label the following structures.

a. _____

b. _____

c. _____

d. _____

e. _____

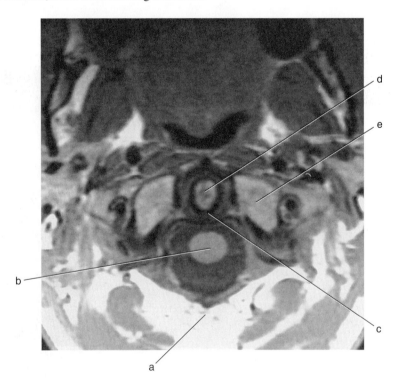

7. On Figure 4.67, axial MRI of the lumbar vertebra, label the following structures.

a. _____

b. _____

c. _____

d. _____

e. _____

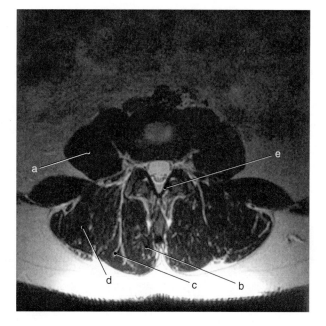

8. On Figure 4.79, axial CT of the thoracic vertebra, label the following structures.

a. _____

b. _____

c. _____

d. _____

e. _____

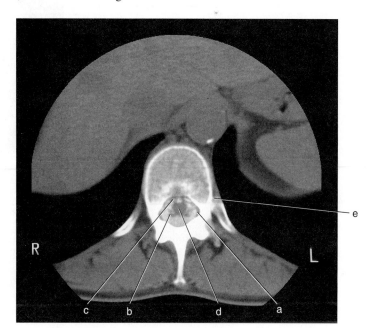

9. On Figure 4.41, midsagittal MRI of cervical spine demonstrating spinal ligaments, label the following structures.

a. _____

b. _____

c. _____

d. _____

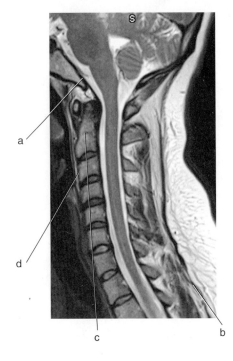

10. On Figure 4.109, coronal MRI of spine, label the following structures.

a. _____

b. _____

c. _____

d. _____

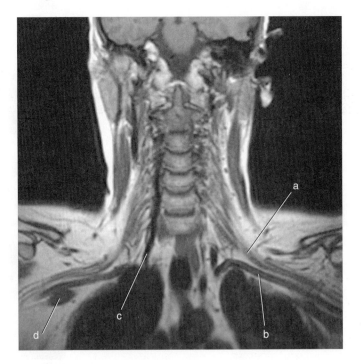

11. On Figure 4.85, sagittal MRI of lumbar spine, label the following structures.

a. _____

b. _____

c. _____

d. _____

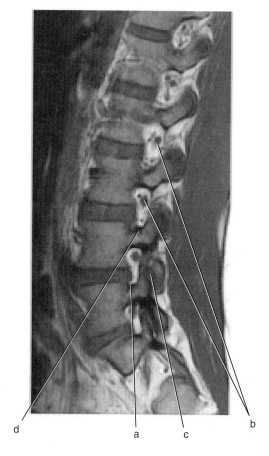

12. On Figure 4.15, coronal MRI of cervical spine, label the following structures.

a. _____

b. _____

c. _____

d. _____

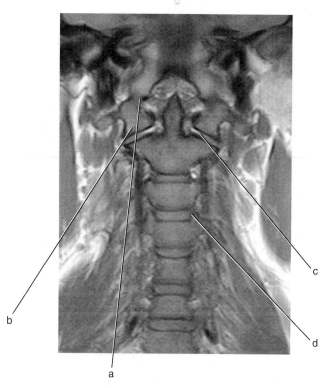

13. On Figure 4.18, sagittal CT reformat of C1 and C2, label the following structures.

a. _____

b. _____

c. _____

d. _____

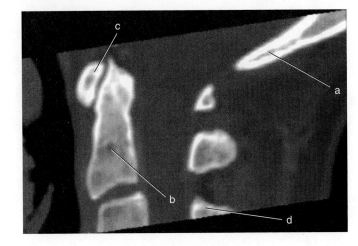

14. On Figure 4.25, midsagittal MRI of cervical and thoracic spines, label the following structures.

a. _____

b. _____

c. _____

d. _____

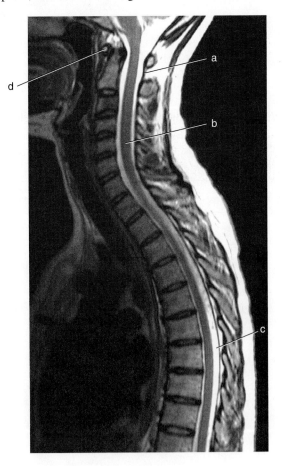

15. On Figure 4.42, sagittal CT reformat of atlantooccipital joint, label the following structures.

a. _____

b. _____

c. _____

d. _____

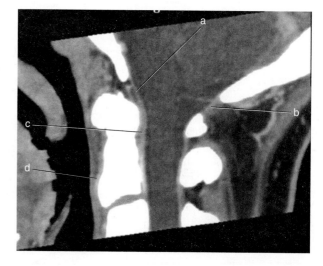

16. On Figure 4.20, 3D CT of cervical vertebrae, label the following structures.

a. _____

b. _____

c. _____

d. _____

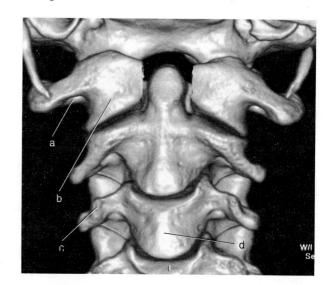

17. On Figure 4.80, axial MRI of lumbar vertebra, label the following structures.

a. _____

b. _____

c. _____

d. _____

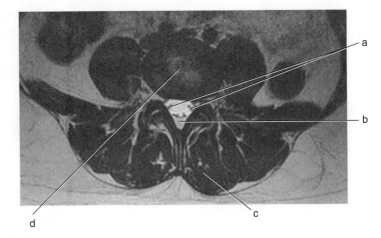

18. On Figure 4.105, sagittal oblique MRI oblique of cervical plexus, label the following structures.

a. _____

b. _____

c. _____

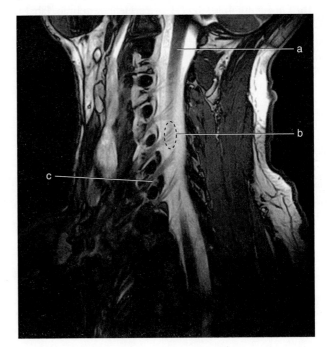

19. On Figure 4.114, sagittal MRI scan of brachial plexus, label the following structures.

    a. _____

    b. _____

    c. _____

    d. _____

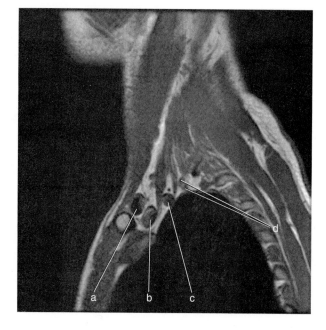

20. On Figure 4.29, coronal CT reformat of thoracic spine, post myelogram, label the following structures.

    a. _____

    b. _____

    c. _____

    d. _____

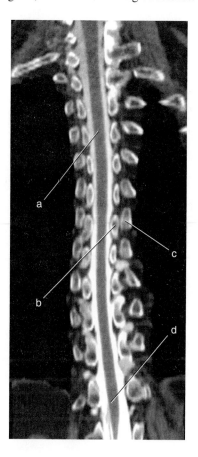

Chapter **4** **Spine**

21. On Figure 4.30, 3D CT of lumbar spine, anterior view, label the following structures.

a. _____

b. _____

c. _____

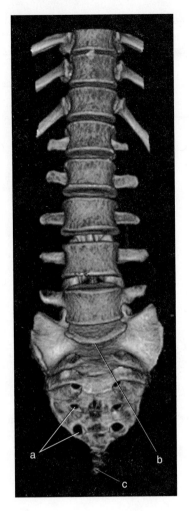

22. On Figure 4.49, midsagittal, MRI of lumbar spine with spinal ligaments, label the following structures.

a. _____

b. _____

c. _____

d. _____

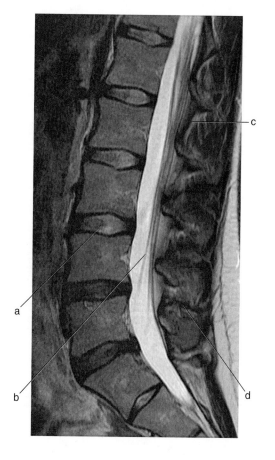

23. On Figure 4.60, axial MRI of thoracic vertebra with spinal muscles, label the following structures.

a. _____

b. _____

c. _____

d. _____

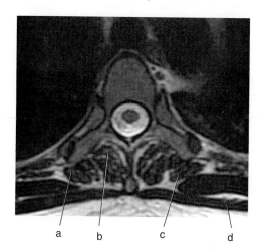

24. On Figure 4.57, axial CT of cervical vertebra with spinal muscles, label the following structures.

a. _____

b. _____

c. _____

d. _____

e. _____

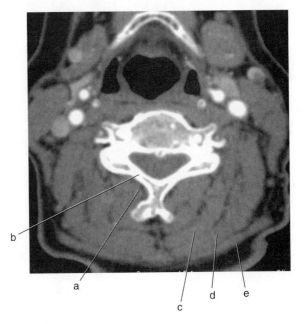

25. On Figure 4.77, coronal CT reformat of spinal cord, label the following structures.

a. _____

b. _____

c. _____

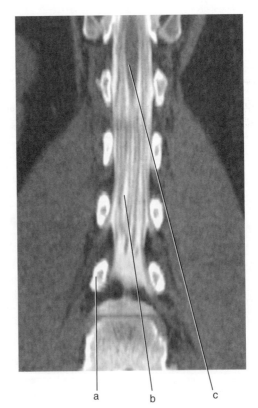

26. On Figure 4.113, coronal MRI of cervical spine, label the following structures.

a. _____

b. _____

c. _____

d. _____

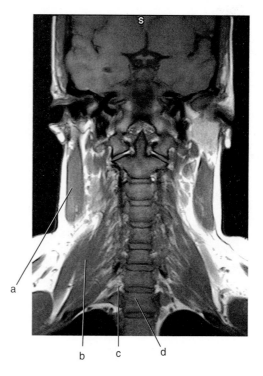

27. On Figure 4.120, coronal MRI of sacroiliac joints, label the following structures.

a. _____

b. _____

c. _____

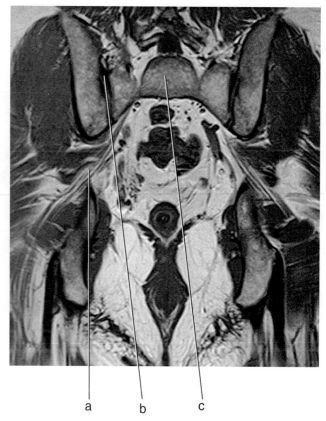

28. On Figure 4.131, 3D CT of lumbar spine, anterior oblique view, label the following structures.

a. _____

b. _____

c. _____

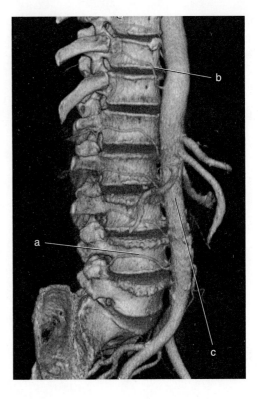

29. On Figure 4.136, axial MRI of lumbar vertebra, label the following structures.

a. _____

b. _____

c. _____

d. _____

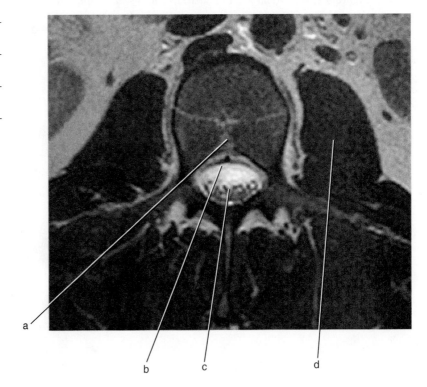

30. On Figure 4.63, coronal CT reformat of lumbar vertebrae with spinal muscles, label the following structures.

a. _____

b. _____

c. _____

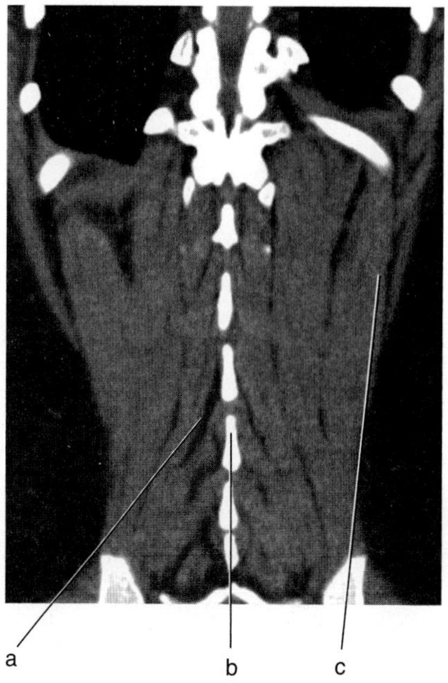

a   b   c

CASE STUDIES

Case Study 1

A 16-year-old male who had a diving accident received a cervical spine CT that revealed a Jefferson fracture. A Jefferson fracture is a burst type fracture that occurs at the anterior and posterior arches of C1 (atlas).

1. Describe the anatomy of C1.

2. Approximately one third of these fractures are associated with an axis fracture. Describe the axis and its articulation with the atlas.

3. Why would vertebral artery injuries possibly occur as a result of a Jefferson fracture?

Case Study 2

A 56-year-old female experiencing neck pain received a cervical MRI that demonstrated cervical intervertebral disk herniations at C3-C4 and C7-T1.

1. Describe the anatomy and function of the intervertebral disk.

2. What is an intervertebral disk herniation?

5 | Neck

OBJECTIVES

1. List the three anatomic sections of the pharynx.
2. List and identify the laryngeal cartilages.
3. Identify and describe the esophagus and trachea.
4. Identify and state the function of the salivary glands.
5. Describe the location and function of the thyroid gland.
6. List the cervical lymph node regions.
7. Identify the fascial planes and spaces.
8. Identify the pharyngeal muscles.
9. State the triangles of the neck and identify the muscles that divide them.
10. Describe the course of the major vessels located within the neck.

After reading Chapter 5, see if you can complete the following problems.

MATCHING

Match each muscle to its correct descriptor.

1. _____ Genioglossus muscle
2. _____ Platysma muscle
3. _____ SCM
4. _____ Constrictor muscles
5. _____ Suprahyoid muscles
6. _____ Infrahyoid muscles
7. _____ Trapezius muscle
8. _____ Splenius capitis muscle
9. _____ Scalene muscles

a. One of the extrinsic muscles responsible for changing the position of the tongue
b. Changes facial expression
c. Often called strap muscles because of their ribbon-like appearance
d. Inserts on the occipital bone and acts to extend the head
e. Straplike muscle that originates on the sternum and clavicle and inserts on the mastoid tip of the temporal bone
f. A superficial muscle located on the posterior portion of the neck that acts to elevate the scapula
g. Responsible for constricting the pharynx and inducing peristaltic waves during swallowing
h. Elevates the hyoid bone and floor of the mouth and tongue during swallowing and speaking
i. Act to elevate the upper two ribs and flex the neck

MULTIPLE CHOICE

1. Which of the following is considered the smallest of the salivary glands?
   a. Parotid
   b. Sublingual
   c. Submaxillary
   d. Submandibular

2. The thyroid gland is located at the level of the:
   a. Thyroid cartilage
   b. Manubrium
   c. Hyoid bone
   d. Cricoid cartilage

3. How many cartilages make up the larynx?
   a. Three pairs
   b. Six pairs
   c. 9
   d. 12

4. Foreign objects can commonly become lodged in the:
   a. Uvula
   b. Thyroid cartilage
   c. Valleculae
   d. Arytenoid cartilage

5. The brachial plexus is located between the:
   a. Platysma and posterior scalene muscles
   b. Middle and posterior scalene muscles
   c. Sternocleidomastoid and anterior scalene muscles
   d. Anterior and middle scalene muscles

6. Which of the following is typically the largest vascular structure located in the neck?
   a. Common carotid artery
   b. Internal jugular vein
   c. Internal carotid artery
   d. External jugular vein

7. Which muscle covers most of the anterior surface of the neck?
   a. Trapezius
   b. Platysma
   c. Scalene
   d. Pterygoid

8. Which cartilage is the epiglottis attached to?
   a. Thyroid
   b. Arytenoid
   c. Cricoid
   d. Hyoid

9. Which muscle divides the neck into anterior and posterior triangles?
   a. Trapezius
   b. Platysma
   c. Longissimus dorsi
   d. Sternocleidomastoid

10. What is the function of the hyoid bone?
    a. Acts as an attachment site for muscles associated with swallowing
    b. Prevents food from entering the trachea
    c. Protects the delicate vocal cords
    d. Acts as a base for the laryngeal cartilages to rest on

FILL IN THE BLANKS

Fill in the blank spaces in the following sentences.

1. The _____ is a small pear-shaped cavity located on each side of the opening to the larynx.

2. The largest and most superior cartilage making up the larynx is the _____.

3. The common carotid artery bifurcates at the level of _____.

4. The vocal cords are best imaged during _____ breathing.

5. Another name for the false vocal cords is the _____.

6. The _____ cartilage forms the base of the larynx.

7. In the roof and posterior wall of the nasopharynx is a collection of lymphoid tissue, known as the _____.

8. The _____ is the space between the true and false vocal cords.

9. The esophagus enters the abdominal cavity to join the stomach through an opening in the diaphragm termed the _____.

10. The suprahyoid and infrahyoid regions of the neck can be further divided by _____ that separate the anatomy of each region into compartments or spaces that contain distinct anatomic structures.

FILL IN THE TABLE

Write in an answer next to the "x" in the following table.

Arteries of the Neck (see Table 5.4)	Origin	Branches
Common carotid artery Left common carotid Right common carotid	 x _____ Right brachiocephalic artery	x _____
x _____	Common carotid artery	Ophthalmic, anterior, and middle cerebral arteries
External carotid artery	x _____	Superior thyroid, lingual, facial, occipital, posterior auricular, and ascending pharyngeal arteries
Vertebral arteries (unite to form basilar artery)	Subclavian artery	x _____

Veins of the Neck (see Table 5.5)	Termination	Tributaries
Internal jugular vein	x _____	Inferior petrosal sinus, facial, lingual, pharyngeal, superior and middle thyroid, and occasionally the occipital veins
External jugular vein	x _____	Retromandibular, anterior jugular, temporal, maxillary veins, and occasionally the occipital vein
x _____	Brachiocephalic vein	Internal and external vertebral venous plexuses and deep cervical veins

TRUE/FALSE

Circle either True or False for each of the following statements.

True/False   1. The cricoid cartilage is a paired cartilage of the larynx.

True/False   2. The external carotid artery passes through the parotid gland as it ascends the neck.

True/False   3. The true vocal cords are located superior to the false vocal cords.

True/False   4. The trachea is reinforced by many C-shaped pieces of cartilage.

True/False   5. The carotid sheath encloses the external jugular vein.

True/False   6. The larynx extends from approximately the third to the sixth cervical vertebrae.

True/False   7. The corniculate cartilages are involved in the movement of the vocal cords for the production of sound.

True/False   8. The submandibular duct is also referred to as Rivinus's duct.

True/False   9. Approximately 40 to 50 sublingual ducts open in a line along the floor of the mouth.

True/False   10. The lymph nodes of the neck can be classified or divided into seven levels or regions for ease of identification, both clinically and surgically.

SHORT ANSWER

1. Describe the location of the oropharynx.

2. List the three paired cartilages of the larynx.

3. The internal jugular veins drain blood from which parts of the body?

4. From which artery does the right common carotid artery arise?

5. Describe the location of the parotid gland.

6. Why does the parotid gland's appearance differ from the other salivary glands?

7. List two hormones that are excreted by the thyroid gland.

1. On Figure 5.4, midsagittal MRI of pharyngeal divisions, label the following structures.

   a. _____

   b. _____

   c. _____

   d. _____

   e. _____

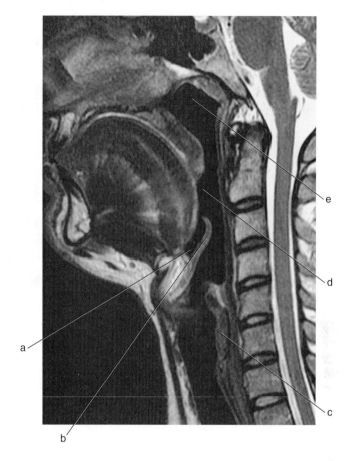

2. On Figure 5.5, sagittal CT reformat of pharynx, label the following structures.

   a. _____

   b. _____

   c. _____

   d. _____

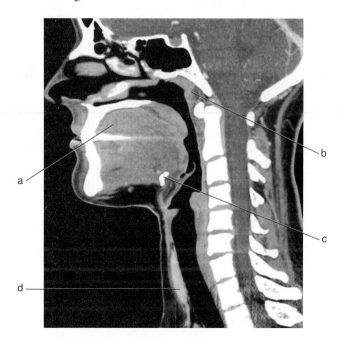

3. On Figure 5.11, axial CT of the neck with oropharynx, label the following structures.

a. _____

b. _____

c. _____

d. _____

e. _____

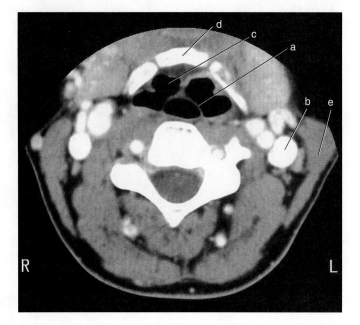

4. On Figure 5.25, axial CT of neck, label the following structures.

a. _____

b. _____

c. _____

d. _____

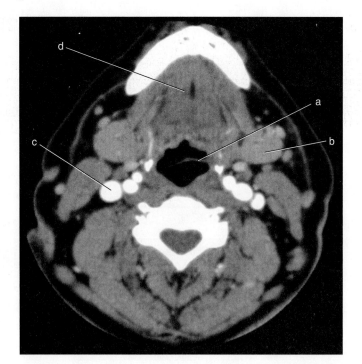

5. On Figure 5.65, axial CT of neck, label the following structures.

a. _____

b. _____

c. _____

d. _____

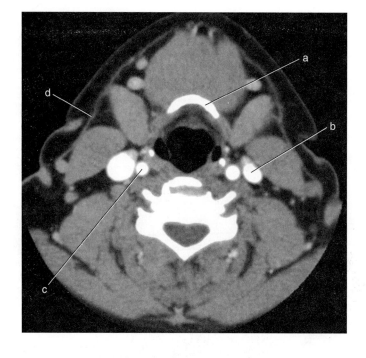

6. On Figure 5.67, axial CT of neck, label the following structures.

a. _____

b. _____

c. _____

d. _____

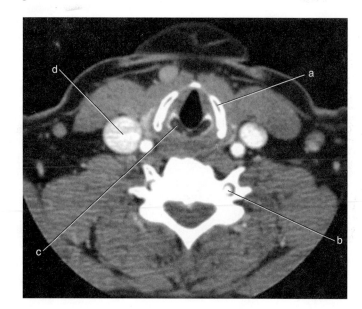

7. On Figure 5.48, axial CT of neck, label the following structures.

a. _____

b. _____

c. _____

d. _____

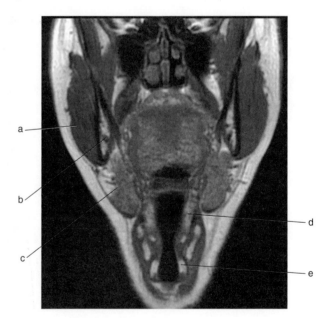

8. On Figure 5.13, coronal MRI of larynx, label the following structures.

a. _____

b. _____

c. _____

d. _____

e. _____

9. On Figure 5.15, coronal CT reformat of neck, label the following structures.

a. _____

b. _____

c. _____

d. _____

e. _____

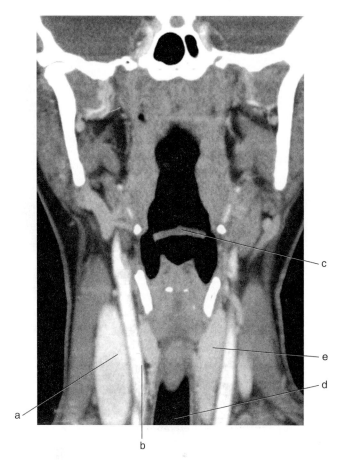

10. On Figure 5.14, coronal CT reformat of neck, label the following structures.

a. _____

b. _____

c. _____

d. _____

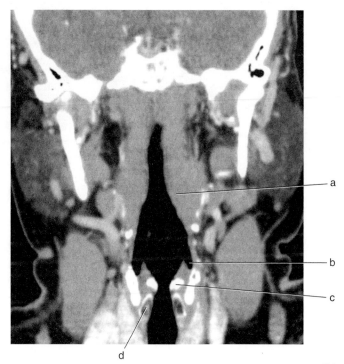

11. On Figure 5.38, coronal MRI of neck, label the following structures.

    a. _____

    b. _____

    c. _____

    d. _____

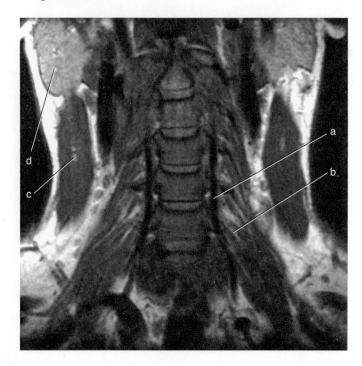

12. On Figure 5.36, axial MRI of neck, label the following structures.

    a. _____

    b. _____

    c. _____

    d. _____

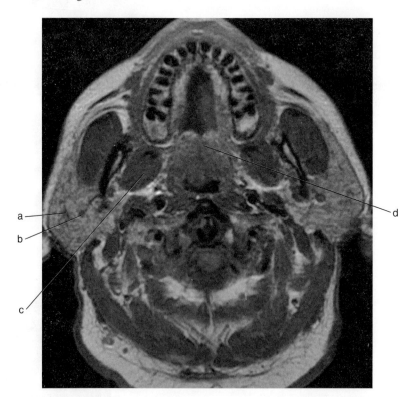

13. On Figure 5.43, axial MRI of neck, label the following structures.

a. _____

b. _____

c. _____

d. _____

e. _____

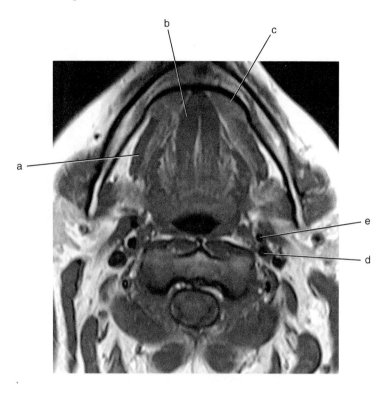

14. On Figure 5.10, axial MRI of neck, label the following structures.

a. _____

b. _____

c. _____

d. _____

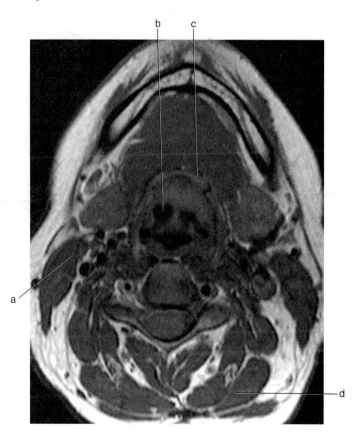

15. On Figure 5.64, axial MRI of neck with hyoid bone, label the following structures.

    a. _____

    b. _____

    c. _____

    d. _____

    e. _____

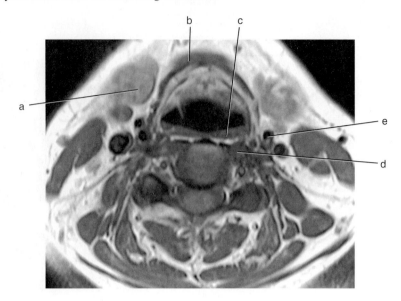

16. On Figure 5.24, axial MRI of neck with epiglottis, label the following structures.

    a. _____

    b. _____

    c. _____

    d. _____

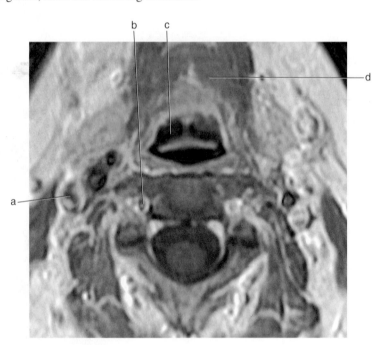

17. On Figure 5.26, axial MRI of larynx, label the following structures.

a. _____

b. _____

c. _____

d. _____

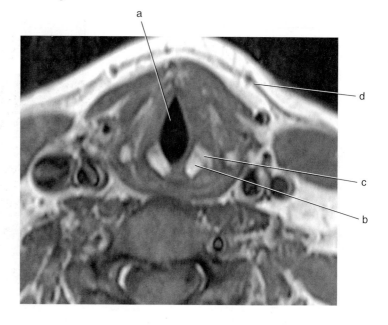

18. On Figure 5.28, axial MRI of larynx, label the following structures.

a. _____

b. _____

c. _____

d. _____

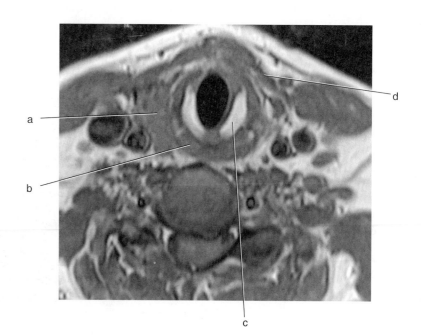

19. On Figure 5.16, axial MRI of laryngopharynx, label the following structures.

a. _____

b. _____

c. _____

d. _____

e. _____

f. _____

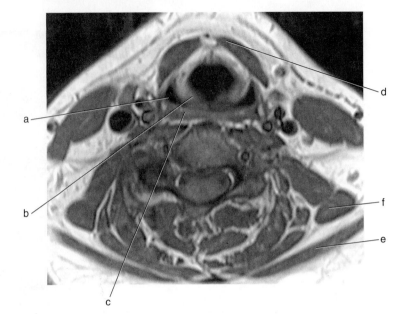

20. On Figure 5.68, axial MRI of neck, label the following structures.

a. _____

b. _____

c. _____

d. _____

e. _____

f. _____

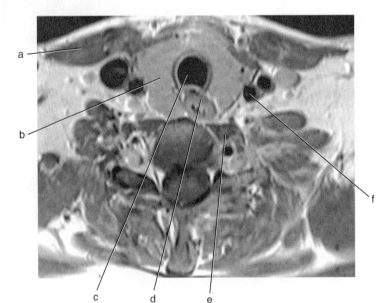

21. On Figure 5.85, 3D CTA of intracranial and extracranial arteries, label the following structures.

a. _____

b. _____

c. _____

d. _____

e. _____

f. _____

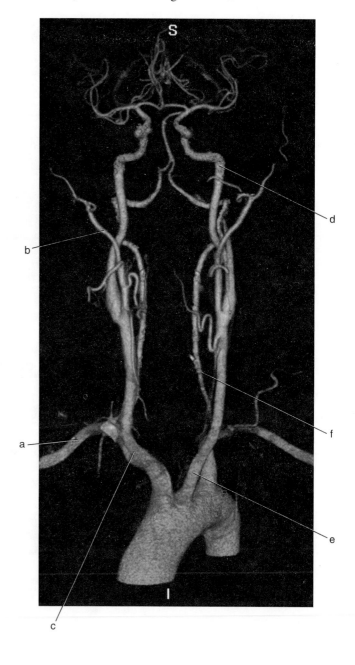

22. On Figure 5.84, MRA of extracranial arteries, label the following structures.

a. _____

b. _____

c. _____

d. _____

e. _____

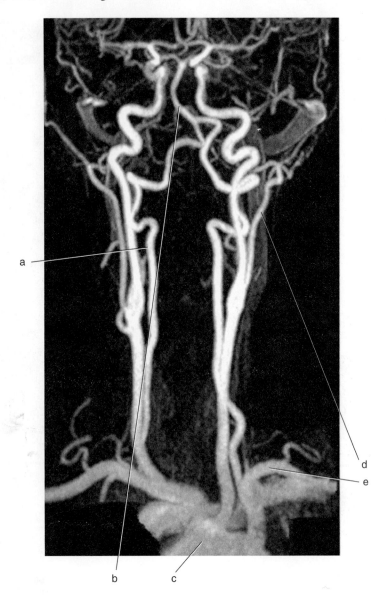

23. On Figure 5.83, anterior oblique 3D CTA of extracranial arteries, label the following structures.

a. _____

b. _____

c. _____

d. _____

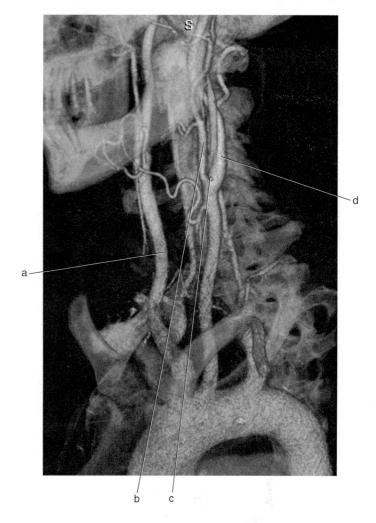

Case Study 1

A 25-year-old man presented with an enlarging mass in the right cervical region of the neck. The mass was soft but nontender. A contrast-enhanced CT demonstrated a fluid-filled cystic mass adjacent to the larynx, representing a laryngocele.

1. What cartilages make up the larynx?

2. What important structures are located within the larynx?

Case Study 2

A 38-year-old female was involved in a snow skiing accident. She presented to the ER with complaints of a left-sided headache, neck pain, and pulsatile tinnitus. An MRI demonstrated abnormal increased signal intensity surrounding the left internal carotid artery, due to a dissection of the vessel.

1. What level does the common carotid bifurcate into the internal and external carotid arteries?

2. What is the dilatation found at the origin of the internal carotid artery called?

6 | Thorax

OBJECTIVES

1. Describe the structures that comprise the bony thorax.
2. Define the thoracic inlet and outlet.
3. Understand the function and layers of the pleura.
4. Identify and describe the structures of the lungs.
5. Identify the mainstem bronchi and their divisions.
6. List the structures of the mediastinum, and describe their anatomic relationships to each other.
7. Identify the structures of the heart, and explain the circulation of blood through the heart.
8. Identify the great vessels, and describe the distribution of their associated arteries and veins.
9. Differentiate between pulmonary arteries and veins by function and location.
10. Identify the coronary arteries and veins.
11. List the muscles involved with respiration by function and location.

After reading Chapter 6, see if you can complete the following problems.

MULTIPLE CHOICE

1. The aorta arises from the:
   a. Right atrium
   b. Left atrium
   c. Right ventricle
   d. Left ventricle

2. The pulmonary veins bring blood to the:
   a. Right atrium
   b. Left atrium
   c. Right ventricle
   d. Left ventricle

3. The first vessel to branch off the aortic arch is the:
   a. Brachiocephalic artery
   b. Left common carotid artery
   c. Left subclavian artery
   d. Left vertebral artery

4. Which of the following is the chief muscle of respiration?
   a. Intercostals
   b. Diaphragm
   c. Rhomboid
   d. Serratus

5. The superior vena cava is formed by the junction of the:
   a. Internal jugular veins
   b. External jugular veins
   c. Subclavian veins
   d. Brachiocephalic veins

6. Which of the following makes up the apex of the heart?
   a. Right atrium
   b. Left atrium
   c. Right ventricle
   d. Left ventricle

7. Collateral circulation between the inferior vena cava and the superior vena cava is supplied by the:
   a. Thoracic veins
   b. Subclavian veins
   c. Azygos veins
   d. Intercostal veins

8. Which of the following is not considered a mediastinal structure?
   a. Heart
   b. Lungs
   c. Trachea
   d. Thymus gland

9. The thickest, strongest muscle in the heart is located in the:
   a. Right atrium
   b. Left atrium
   c. Right ventricle
   d. Left ventricle

10. Which of the following is located between the upper thoracic vertebrae and trachea?
    a. Aorta
    b. Esophagus
    c. Thoracic duct
    d. Azygos vein

FILL IN THE BLANKS

Fill in the blank spaces in the following sentences.

1. The heart is lined by a serous membrane called the

   _____.

2. The _____ is the middle muscular layer of the heart wall.

3. The _____ is the area where vessels and nerves enter and exit the lungs.

4. The four _____ bring oxygenated blood to the left atrium.

5. _____ is located between the pericardium and the heart wall and is most prominent around the inflow and outflow of the heart.

6. Another name for the medial angle of the lung is the

   _____.

7. The _____ supplies blood to the right atrium and right ventricle of the heart.

8. Within the mediastinum, clusters of _____ are clumped around the great vessels, esophagus, bronchi, and carina.

9. The aperture known as the _____ allows for the passage of nerves, vessels, and viscera from the neck into the thoracic cavity.

10. The lateral angle of the lung is termed the

    _____.

11. Deep pockets or recesses of the pleural cavities are the costomediastinal and _____ recesses.

12. The secondary bronchi further divide into the _____.

13. The diaphragm is attached to the lumbar spine via two tendinous structures termed _____.

14. The _____ layer of the breast consists of glandular tissue, excretory ducts, and connective tissues.

15. The thymus gland produces a hormone, _____, which is responsible for the development and maturation of lymphocytes.

MATCHING

Match each structure to its corresponding feature.

_____ 1. Aortic valve
_____ 2. Myocardium
_____ 3. Tricuspid valve
_____ 4. Hilum
_____ 5. Windpipe
_____ 6. Serratus anterior muscle
_____ 7. Diaphragm
_____ 8. Azygos vein
_____ 9. Levatores costarum muscle
_____ 10. Cooper's ligaments
_____ 11. Visceral pleura
_____ 12. Pulmonary arteries

a. Laterally rotate and protract scapula
b. Opening on medial surface of the lungs
c. Cords of connective tissue
d. Elevates the ribs
e. Middle layer of heart wall
f. Semilunar valve
g. Right atrioventricular valve
h. Collateral circulation
i. Covers lung surface
j. Carries deoxygenated blood to lungs
k. Chief muscle of respiration
l. Trachea

HEART MAP

Using the terms below, match the numbers on the drawing to their corresponding terms.

_____ Aortic semilunar valve
_____ Pulmonary semilunar valve
_____ Bicuspid valve
_____ Tricuspid valve
_____ Aorta
_____ Left common carotid artery
_____ Pulmonary veins
_____ Pulmonary arteries
_____ Inferior vena cava
_____ Superior vena cava
_____ Brachiocephalic artery
_____ Interventricular septum
_____ Right atrium
_____ Left atrium
_____ Right ventricle
_____ Left ventricle
_____ Left subclavian artery

SHORT ANSWER

1. List six structures located within the mediastinum.

2. Describe the primary function of the thymus gland.

3. What areas of the body does the thoracic duct drain?

4. Describe how blood enters the heart, is circulated through the heart, and then exits the heart.

5. Describe how the short axis (SA) view can be obtained.

6. List the three main branches of the aortic arch.

7. List the tributaries of the superior vena cava.

8. Describe the coronary sinus.

9. What is the function of the azygos venous system?

10. List the three layers of breast tissue.

TRUE/FALSE

Circle either True or False for each of the following statements.

True/False   1. The inferior lobe of the right lung is separated from the middle and superior lobes by the horizontal fissure.

True/False   2. Each lung has an opening on its medial surface termed the hilum.

True/False   3. The visceral pleura, the outer layer of the pleura, is continuous with the thoracic wall and diaphragm and moves with these structures during respiration.

True/False   4. The trachea bifurcates into the left and right mainstem bronchi at approximately the level of T10.

True/False   5. The inner surface of the fibrous pericardium consists of a double-layered serous membrane termed the serous pericardium.

True/False   6. During embryonic development an oval opening exists within the interatrial septum called the foramen ovale.

True/False   7. The pulmonary semilunar valve is located at the juncture of the left ventricle and pulmonary trunk.

True/False   8. The left pulmonary artery is shorter and smaller than the right pulmonary artery and is the most superior of the pulmonary vessels.

True/False   9. The right superior pulmonary vein passes anterior and inferior to the right pulmonary artery.

True/False   10. The right coronary artery arises from the base or root of the aorta.

FILL IN THE TABLE (see Table 6.6)

Fill in the blanks in the following table.

Muscles of the Anterior and Lateral Walls of the Thorax

Muscle	Origin	Insertion	Action
Pectoralis major	Clavicular head—medial half of clavicle. Sternal head—lateral manubrium and sternum, six upper costal cartilages	_____	_____
Pectoralis minor	Anterior surface of ribs 3-5	_____	Elevates ribs of scapula, protracts scapula, and assists serratus anterior
_____	First rib and cartilage	Inferior surface of the clavicle	Depresses the shoulder and assists pectoralis in inspiration
Serratus anterior	Angles of superior 8-9 ribs	Medial border of scapula	_____

IDENTIFY

1. On Figure 6.12, coronal CT reformat of lungs, label the following structures.

   a. _____

   b. _____

   c. _____

   d. _____

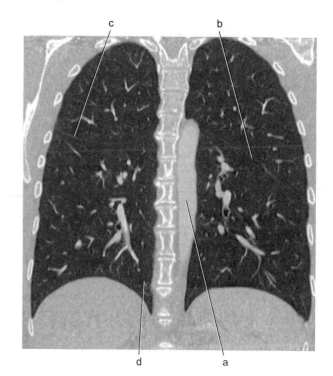

2. On Figure 6.18, axial CT of chest, label the following structures.

a. _____

b. _____

c. _____

d. _____

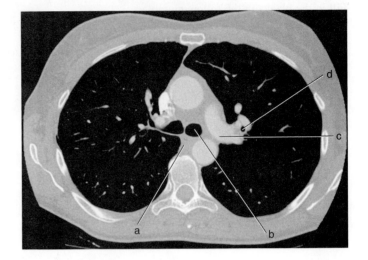

3. On Figure 6.38, coronal MRI of the heart, label the following structures.

a. _____

b. _____

c. _____

d. _____

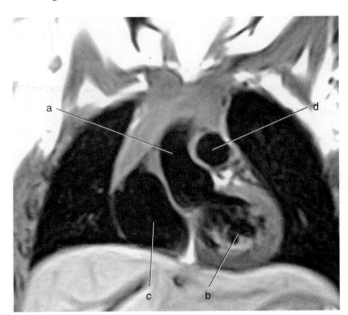

4. On Figure 6.49, axial CT of heart, label the following structures.

a. _____

b. _____

c. _____

d. _____

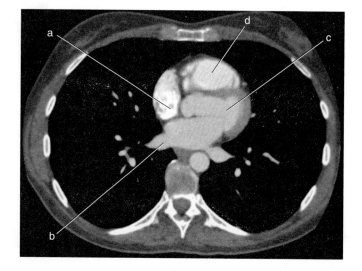

5. On Figure 6.93, sagittal MRI of inferior vena cava, label the following structures.

a. _____

b. _____

c. _____

d. _____

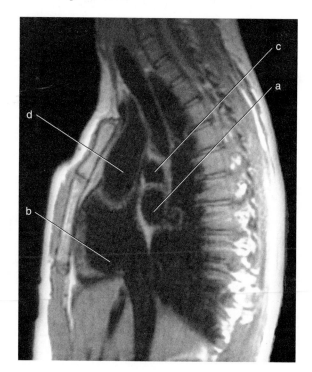

6. On Figure 6.99, axial CT of chest, label the following structures.

a. _____

b. _____

c. _____

d. _____

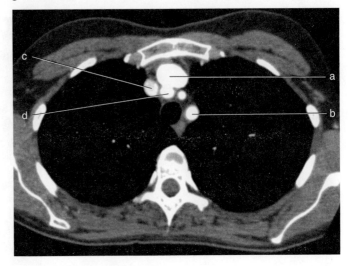

7. On Figure 6.144, axial CT of chest, label the following structures.

a. _____

b. _____

c. _____

d. _____

e. _____

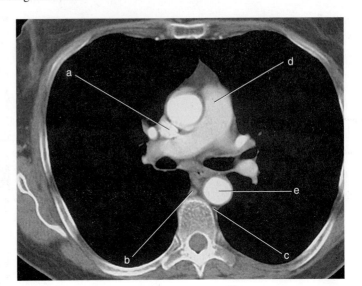

8. On Figure 6.159, sagittal MRI of female breast, label the following structures.

    a. _____

    b. _____

    c. _____

    d. _____

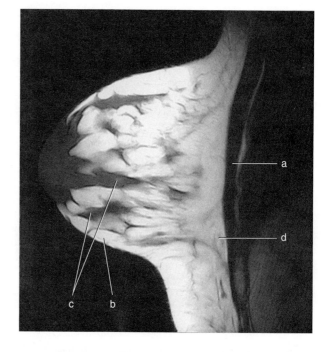

9. On Figure 6.47, axial CT of heart, label the following structures.

    a. _____

    b. _____

    c. _____

    d. _____

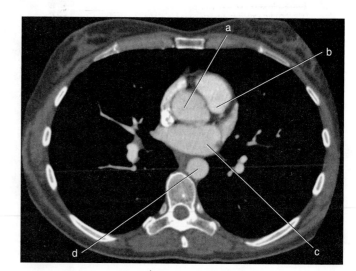

10. On Figure 6.52, axial MRI of heart, label the following structures.

a. _____

b. _____

c. _____

d. _____

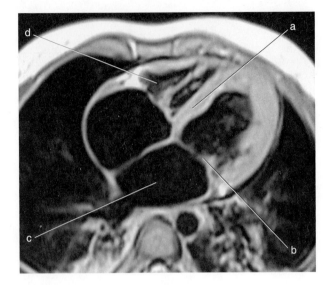

11. On Figure 6.80, coronal CT reformat of chest, label the following structures.

a. _____

b. _____

c. _____

d. _____

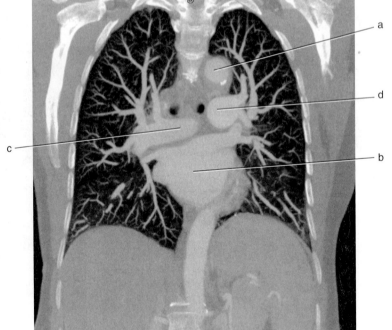

12. On Figure 6.91, sagittal MRI of left mediastinum, label the following structures.

a. _____

b. _____

c. _____

d. _____

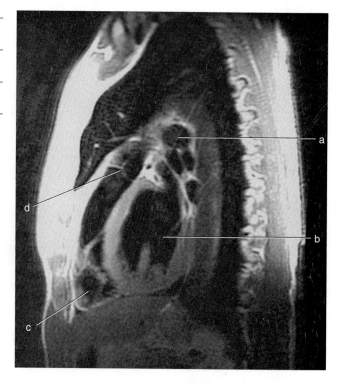

13. On Figure 6.101, pulmonary MRA, label the following structures.

a. _____

b. _____

c. _____

d. _____

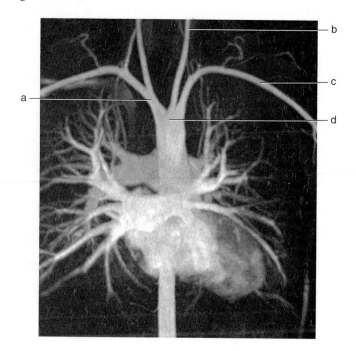

14. On Figure 6.104, axial MRA of heart, label the following structures.

a. _____

b. _____

c. _____

d. _____

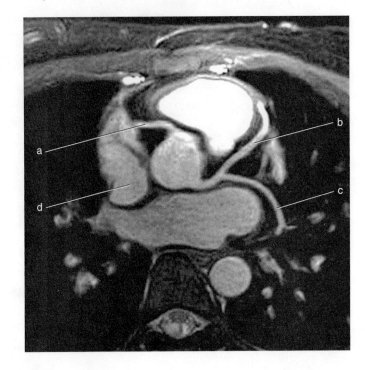

15. On Figure 6.106, MRA of heart, label the following structures.

a. _____

b. _____

c. _____

d. _____

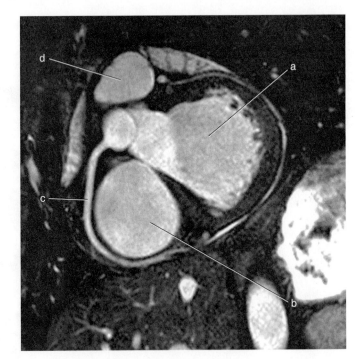

16. On Figure 6.109, axial MRA of heart, label the following structures.

a. _____

b. _____

c. _____

d. _____

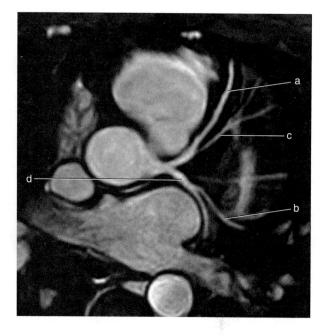

17. On Figure 6.24, axial CT of secondary pulmonary lobule, label the following structures.

a. _____

b. _____

c. _____

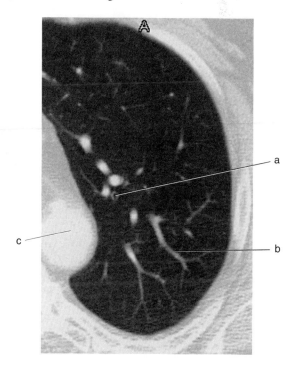

18. On Figure 6.29, axial MRI of chest, label the following structures.

a. _____

b. _____

c. _____

d. _____

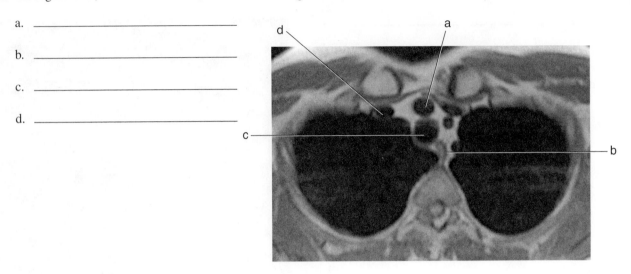

19. On Figure 6.122, vertical long axis CT, label the following structures.

a. _____

b. _____

c. _____

d. _____

20. On Figure 6.152, coronal CT reformat of chest, label the following structures.

a. _____

b. _____

c. _____

d. _____

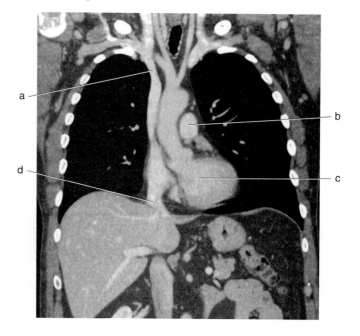

21. On Figure 6.50, axial MRI of right atrium, label the following structures.

a. _____

b. _____

c. _____

d. _____

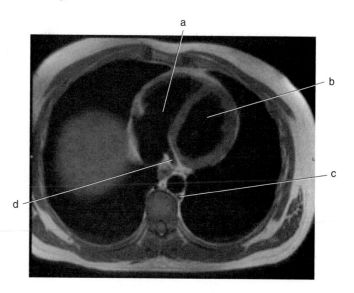

22. On Figure 6.61, sagittal CT reformat of heart, label the following structures.

a. _____

b. _____

c. _____

d. _____

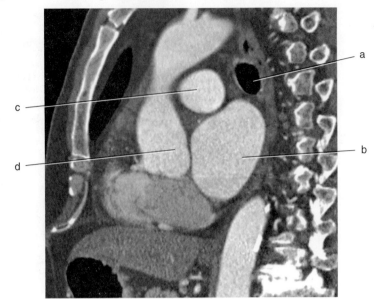

23. On Figure 6.76, pulmonary 3D CTA, posterior view, label the following structures.

a. _____

b. _____

c. _____

d. _____

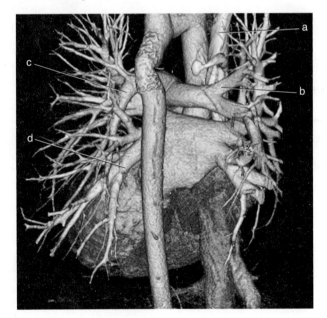

24. On Figure 6.79, pulmonary MRA, label the following structures.

a. _____

b. _____

c. _____

d. _____

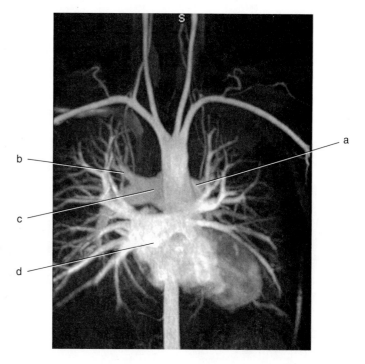

25. On Figure 6.97, 3D CT of aortic arch, label the following structures.

a. _____

b. _____

c. _____

d. _____

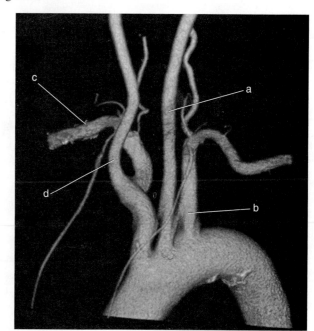

26. On Figure 6.111, 3D CT of heart, label the following structures.

a. _____

b. _____

c. _____

d. _____

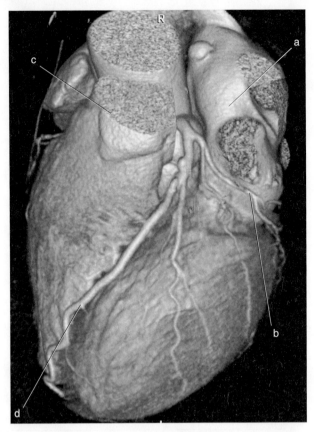

27. On Figure 6.113, axial CT of heart, label the following structures.

a. _____

b. _____

c. _____

d. _____

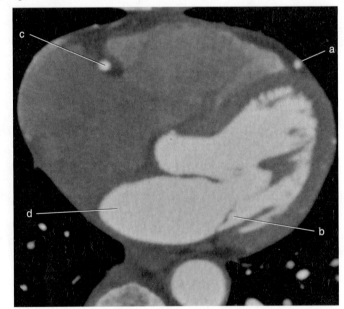

28. On Figure 6.119, 3D CT of heart, label the following structures.

a. _____

b. _____

c. _____

d. _____

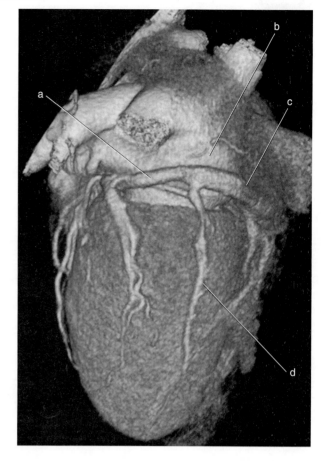

29. On Figure 6.136, right ventricular outflow tract (RVOT) MRI, label the following structures.

a. _____

b. _____

c. _____

d. _____

e. _____

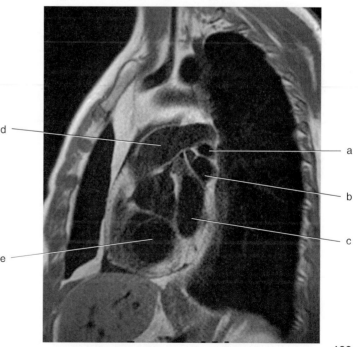

Case Study 1

A 30-year-old female presented to the emergency department complaining of ongoing coldness, numbness, and pain in her right arm. A CT study demonstrated a compression of the right subclavian artery due to a rib anomaly, resulting in thoracic outlet syndrome (a condition involving the thoracic inlet).

1. What structures form the borders of the thoracic inlet or superior thoracic aperture?

2. What structures pass between the neck and the thoracic cavity through the superior thoracic aperture?

Case Study 2

A 40-year-old male developed a progressive cough, chest pain, and dysphagia over the period of one month. A chest radiograph demonstrated a mass in the superior mediastinum, most likely a tumor of the thymus gland (thymoma).

1. What is the function of the thymus gland?

2. Where is the thymus gland located within the thoracic cavity?

7 Abdomen

OBJECTIVES

1. List the structures of the abdominal cavity, and differentiate among those that are contained within the peritoneum and those that are contained within the retroperitoneum.
2. Describe the peritoneal and retroperitoneal spaces.
3. Describe the lobes, segments, and vasculature of the liver.
4. Define the structures of the biliary system.
5. State the functions and location of the pancreas and spleen.
6. Identify the structures of the urinary system.
7. List and identify the structures of the stomach and intestines.
8. Identify the branches of the abdominal aorta and the structures they supply.
9. Identify the tributaries of the inferior vena cava and the structures they drain.
10. List the muscles of the abdomen and describe their function.

After reading Chapter 7, see if you can complete the following problems.

MULTIPLE CHOICE

1. What imaginary line separates the left and right lobes of the liver?
   a. Main lobar fissure
   b. Ligamentum venosum
   c. Falciform ligament
   d. Gerota's fascia

2. What is the largest lobe of the liver?
   a. Right
   b. Left
   c. Quadrate
   d. Caudate

3. The hepatic veins empty into the:
   a. Portal vein
   b. Superior mesenteric vein
   c. Inferior vena cava
   d. Splenic vein

4. Which structure is retroperitoneal?
   a. Gallbladder
   b. Spleen
   c. Pancreas
   d. Stomach

5. Which of the following arteries is not one of the branches of the celiac trunk?
   a. Common hepatic artery
   b. Splenic artery
   c. Left gastric artery
   d. Cystic artery

6. What part of the pancreas is located in the curve of the duodenum?
   a. Head
   b. Neck
   c. Body
   d. Tail

7. What is the smallest lobe of the liver?
   a. Right
   b. Left
   c. Caudate
   d. Quadrate

8. What thin, tendinous structure connects the two rectus abdominis muscles at the midline?
   a. Linea alba
   b. Transversus abdominis
   c. Internal oblique
   d. Ligamentum teres

9. Morison's pouch is located in the:
   a. Subhepatic space
   b. Subphrenic space
   c. Paracolic gutter
   d. Pararenal space

10. Which of the following unite to form the portal vein?
    a. Superior and inferior mesenteric veins
    b. Inferior mesenteric and splenic veins
    c. Superior mesenteric and splenic veins
    d. Splenic and hepatic veins

11. Which of the following ligaments extends from the liver to the anterior abdominal wall and diaphragm and divides the liver anatomically into right and left lobes?
    a. Coronary ligament
    b. Falciform ligament
    c. Round ligament
    d. Gastrophrenic ligament

12. Which of the following spaces is located between the diaphragm and the anterior portion of the liver?
    a. Paracolic gutters
    b. Infracolic spaces
    c. Subhepatic spaces
    d. Subphrenic spaces

13. Current practice favors dividing the liver into how many segments?
    a. 6
    b. 7
    c. 8
    d. 9

14. Which of the following arteries usually arises as one of the three branches of the celiac artery?
    a. Common hepatic artery
    b. Proper hepatic artery
    c. Right hepatic artery
    d. Left hepatic artery

15. Amylase, lipase, and peptidases are enzymes secreted by the:
    a. Liver
    b. Spleen
    c. Pancreas
    d. Adrenal gland

MATCHING

1. _____ Quadratus lumborum muscles

2. _____ Psoas muscles

3. _____ Rectus abdominis muscles

4. _____ Oblique muscles

5. _____ Transverse abdominis muscles

a. Function to flex the lumbar vertebrae and support the abdomen

b. Extend along the lateral surfaces of the lumbar vertebrae

c. Lie deep to the internal oblique muscles and provide maximum support for the abdominal viscera

d. Located on the lateral portion of the abdomen and work together to flex and rotate the vertebral column

e. Form a large portion of the posterior abdominal wall and aid in lateral flexion of the vertebral column

ASSOCIATION

Differentiate between the peritoneal (P) and retro-peritoneal (R) structures by placing the correct letter in front of the structure.

1. _____ Bladder

2. _____ Liver

3. _____ Kidneys

4. _____ Gallbladder

5. _____ Spleen

6. _____ Stomach

7. _____ Pancreas

8. _____ Inferior vena cava

9. _____ Ovaries

10. _____ Prostate gland

11. _____ Duodenum

FILL IN THE BLANKS

Fill in the blank spaces in the following sentences.

1. The liver is surrounded by a strong connective tissue capsule named _____ that gives shape and stability to the soft hepatic tissue.

2. The liver is entirely covered by peritoneum except for the gallbladder fossa and the _____.

3. The right and left hepatic ducts unite at the porta hepatis to form the proximal portion of the _____.

4. The common bile duct follows a groove on the posterior surface of the pancreatic head, then pierces the medial wall of the duodenum along with the _____ through the ampulla of Vater.

5. Located just posterior to the neck of the pancreas is the _____, where the portal vein is formed by the merging of the superior mesenteric and splenic veins.

6. The cellular components of the spleen create a highly vascular, spongy parenchyma called _____ and _____ pulp.

7. The adrenal glands along with the kidneys are enclosed by _____.

8. The renal medulla consists of segments called _____ that radiate from the renal sinus to the outer surface of the kidney.

9. The duodenojejunal flexure is fixed in place by the _____, a suspensory ligament created from the connective tissue around the celiac axis and left crus of the diaphragm.

10. The outer, longitudinal muscle of the large intestine forms three thickened bands called taeniae coli that gather the cecum and colon into a series of pouchlike folds called _____.

113

SHORT ANSWER

1. List the two layers of the peritoneum.

2. The celiac trunk divides into three branches. What are those branches?

3. Describe the location of the superior mesenteric artery, and list the structures it supplies.

4. Describe the mesentery.

5. What is the function of the peritoneal ligaments?

6. List the ligaments that attach the spleen to the greater curvature of the stomach and the left kidney.

7. List the two hormones produced by the adrenal medulla.

8. List the five segments of the kidney.

9. List the structures that form the portal vein.

10. Describe the location of the abdominal lymph nodes.

IDENTIFY

1. On Figure 7.5, axial CT of peritoneal and retroperitoneal structures, label the following structures.

   a. _____

   b. _____

   c. _____

   d. _____

   e. _____

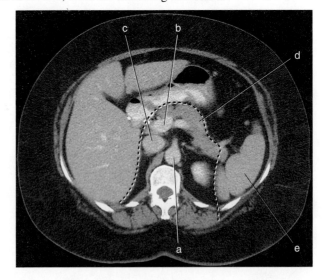

2. On Figure 7.19, axial CT of abdomen, label the following structures.

a. _____

b. _____

c. _____

d. _____

e. _____

f. _____

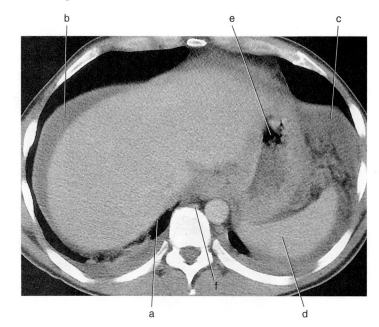

3. On Figure 7.84, axial MRI of abdomen, label the following structures.

a. _____

b. _____

c. _____

d. _____

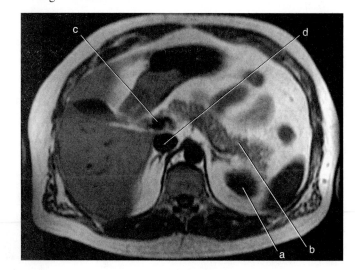

4. On Figure 7.25, axial CT of abdomen, label the following structures.

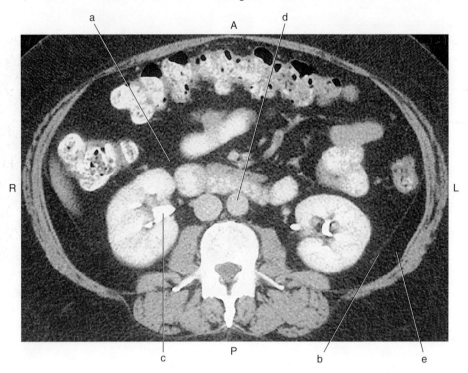

a. _____

b. _____

c. _____

d. _____

e. _____

5. On Figure 7.82, axial MRI of abdomen, label the following structures.

a. _____

b. _____

c. _____

d. _____

e. _____

f. _____

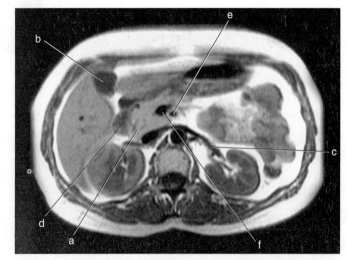

6. On Figure 7.95, axial CT of abdomen, label the following structures.

a. _____

b. _____

c. _____

d. _____

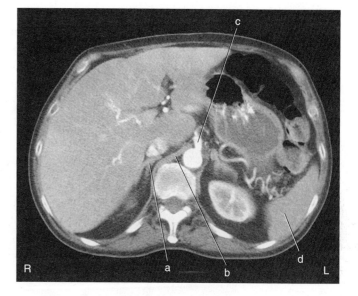

7. On Figure 7.92, coronal MRI of abdomen, label the following structures.

a. _____

b. _____

c. _____

d. _____

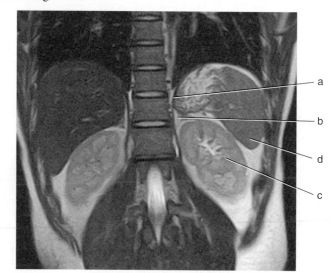

8. On Figure 7.110, axial CT of abdomen, label the following structures.

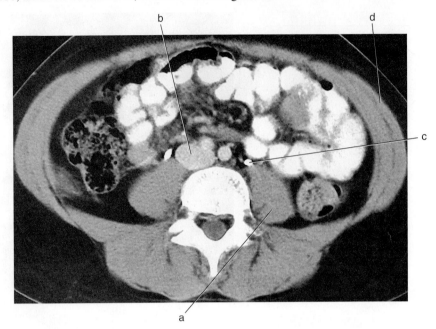

a. _____

b. _____

c. _____

d. _____

9. On Figure 7.152, axial MRI of abdomen, label the following structures.

a. _____

b. _____

c. _____

d. _____

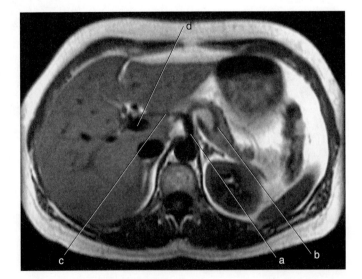

10. On Figure 7.184, axial CT of abdomen, label the following structures.

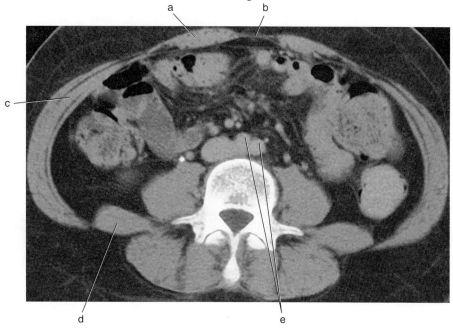

a. _____

b. _____

c. _____

d. _____

e. _____

11. On Figure 7.56, coronal MR venogram of portal system, label the following structures.

a. _____

b. _____

c. _____

d. _____

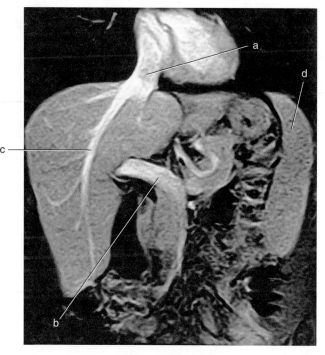

12. On Figure 7.71, MRCP of biliary system, label the following structures.

a. _____

b. _____

c. _____

d. _____

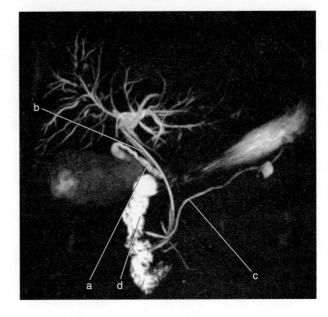

13. On Figure 7.75, axial MRI of abdomen, label the following structures.

a. _____

b. _____

c. _____

d. _____

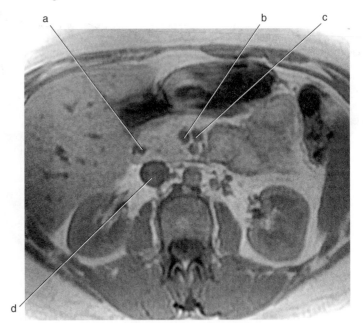

14. On Figure 7.98, axial CT of left adrenal gland, label the following structures.

    a. _____

    b. _____

    c. _____

    d. _____

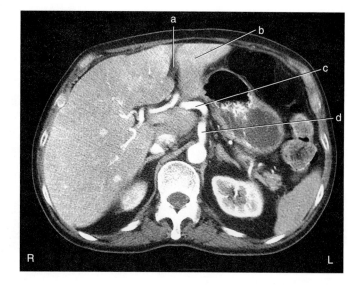

15. On Figure 7.111, 3D CT urogram, label the following structures.

    a. _____

    b. _____

    c. _____

    d. _____

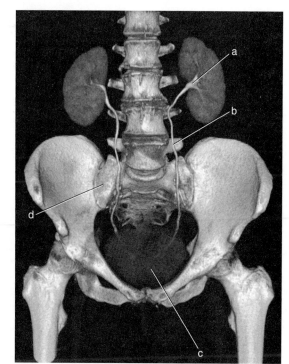

16. On Figure 7.141, 3D CTA of abdominal aorta, label the following structures.

a. _____

b. _____

c. _____

d. _____

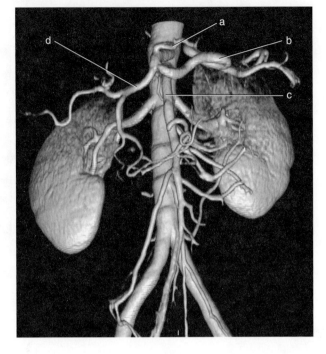

17. On Figure 7.156, MRA of abdominal aorta, label the following structures.

a. _____

b. _____

c. _____

d. _____

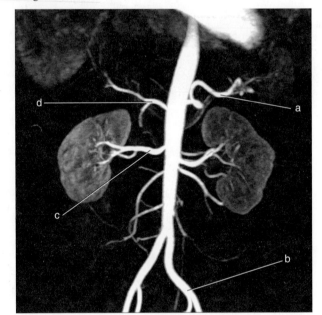

18. On Figure 7.26, coronal MRI of abdomen, label the following structures.

a. _____

b. _____

c. _____

d. _____

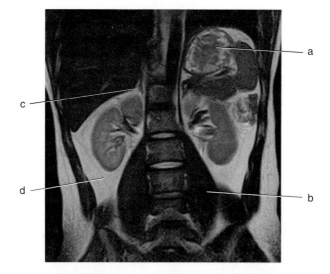

19. On Figure 7.37, coronal CT reformat of liver segments, label the following structures.

a. _____

b. _____

c. _____

d. _____

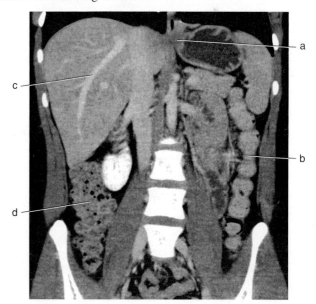

20. On Figure 7.79, axial CT of abdomen, label the following structures.

a. _____

b. _____

c. _____

d. _____

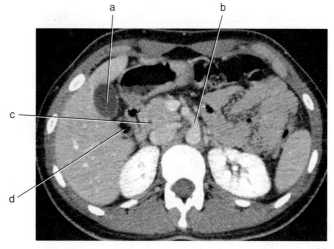

21. On Figure 7.81, sagittal CT reformat of abdomen, label the following structures.

a. _____

b. _____

c. _____

d. _____

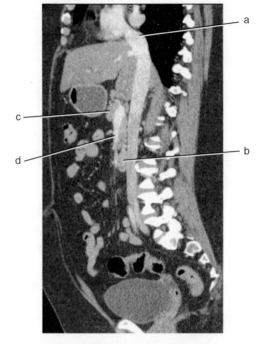

22. On Figure 7.89, axial CT of spleen, label the following structures.

a. _____

b. _____

c. _____

d. _____

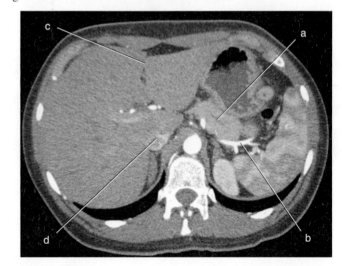

23. On Figure 7.107, axial MRI of kidneys, label the following structures.

a. _____

b. _____

c. _____

d. _____

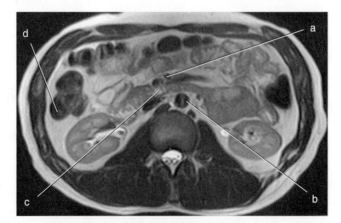

24. On Figure 7.124, axial CT of abdomen, label the following structures.

a. _____

b. _____

c. _____

d. _____

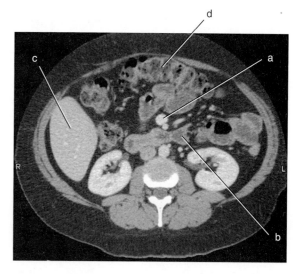

25. On Figure 7.125, coronal CT reformat of small bowel, label the following structures.

a. _____

b. _____

c. _____

d. _____

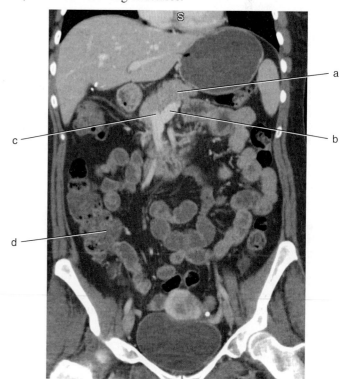

26. On Figure 7.168, 3D CTA of abdominal aorta, label the following structures.

a. _____

b. _____

c. _____

d. _____

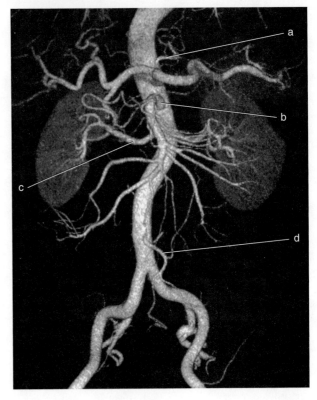

CASE STUDIES

Case Study 1

A 40-year-old male with a history of peptic ulcer disease, presented to the emergency department with a perforation of the ulcer into the supracolic compartment.

1. What is the supracolic compartment and where is it located?

2. What spaces are located within the supracolic compartment?

Case Study 2

A 57-year-old female complained of weight loss, back pain and jaundice for a period of several months. An abdominal CT confirmed a pancreatic adenocarcinoma.

1. Why would jaundice be associated with pancreatic cancer?

2. What is the function of the pancreas?

8 Pelvis

OBJECTIVES

1. Identify the structures of the bony pelvis.
2. Define the pelvic inlet and outlet.
3. Describe the perineum.
4. Describe the function and location of the pelvic muscles.
5. Differentiate between the pelvic and urogenital diaphragms.
6. Describe the location of the bladder in relation to the reproductive organs and the course of the male and female urethras.
7. Describe the location and function of the male and female reproductive organs.
8. Identify the major arteries and veins that are located within the pelvis.
9. Describe the location of the pelvic lymph nodes.

After reading Chapter 8, see if you can complete the following problems.

MULTIPLE CHOICE

1. What is the largest accessory structure of the male reproductive system?
   a. Epididymis
   b. Seminal vesicles
   c. Prostate gland
   d. Spermatic cord

2. Which muscle forms the major part of the pelvic diaphragm?
   a. Obturator internus
   b. Obturator externus
   c. Pectineal
   d. Levator ani

3. The ejaculatory duct opens into the:
   a. Prostatic urethra
   b. Spermatic cord
   c. Penis
   d. Vas deferens

4. What is the largest vein in the body?
   a. Superior vena cava
   b. Inferior vena cava
   c. Left common iliac
   d. Right femoral

5. The male urethra can be divided into how many sections?
   a. One
   b. Two
   c. Three
   d. Four

6. Which broad muscle covers the anterior surface of the iliac fossa?
   a. Piriformis
   b. Iliacus
   c. Obturator internus
   d. Psoas

7. The broad ligament encloses all of the following except:
   a. Ovaries
   b. Uterus
   c. Uterine tubes
   d. Bladder

8. Which structure transports sperm from the testes?
   a. Ejaculatory ducts
   b. Spermatic cords
   c. Vas deferens
   d. Urethra

9. Which of the following acts as a bony landmark separating the abdominal cavity from the pelvic cavity?
   a. Sacroiliac joints
   b. Lateral mass
   c. Iliac fossa
   d. Sacral promontory

10. Which of the following muscles originates from the symphysis pubis and extends to the xyphoid process and costal cartilage of the fifth, sixth, and seventh ribs?
    a. Rectus abdominis
    b. Psoas
    c. External oblique
    d. Internal oblique

11. The muscle that acts to rotate the thigh laterally and originates from the ilium and sacrum and passes through the greater sciatic notch to insert on the greater trochanter of the femur is the:
    a. Obturator internus
    b. Obturator externus
    c. Piriformis
    d. Iliopsoas

12. The muscles that form the posterior portion of the pelvic floor are the:
    a. Levator ani
    b. Coccygeus
    c. Iliopsoas
    d. Obturator

13. Which of the following suspensory ligaments of the uterus help to prevent posterior movement of the uterus as they extend laterally from the uterine cornu through the inguinal canal and anchor to the labia majora?
    a. Uterosacral
    b. Round
    c. Ovarian
    d. Suspensory

14. Which of the following ligaments attach the inferior aspect of the ovaries to the lateral surface of the uterus and uterine tubes?
    a. Ovarian
    b. Suspensory
    c. Uterosacral
    d. Round

15. The obturator and umbilical arteries are branches of which artery?
    a. Internal iliac
    b. External iliac
    c. Common iliac
    d. Deep circumflex iliac

TRUE/FALSE

Circle either True or False for each of the following statements.

True/False   1. The internal and external iliac veins join to form the inferior vena cava.

True/False   2. Sperm are produced in the epididymis.

True/False   3. The round ligaments extend from the cornua of the uterus to prevent posterior movement.

True/False   4. The pectineal line is located on the upper surface of the superior pubic ramus.

True/False   5. The psoas muscle unites with the obturator internus muscle to form the iliopsoas muscle.

True/False   6. The concave, anterior surface of the ala is termed the iliac fossa, which is separated from the body of the ilium by the pectineal line.

True/False   7. An inferior band of fibrous connective tissue from the external oblique muscle folds back on itself to form the inguinal ligament.

True/False   8. The gluteus maximus muscle is the most important muscle for flexing the leg, which makes walking possible.

True/False   9. The posterior surface of the bladder is referred to as the fundus or base.

True/False   10. The apex of the bladder is attached to the anterior abdominal wall by the median umbilical ligament.

MATCHING

Match each of the following phrases to the anatomic structure to which it pertains.

_____ 1. Secretes female sex hormones   a. Prostatic urethra

_____ 2. Protects the fetus   b. Broad ligament

_____ 3. Thickest portion of uterine wall   c. Ovaries

_____ 4. Ejaculatory duct empties into it   d. Vesicouterine pouch

_____ 5. Encloses the ovaries and uterine tubes   e. Vas deferens

_____ 6. Located between the uterus and bladder   f. Membranous urethra

_____ 7. Attaches the ovaries to the pelvic wall   g. Uterus

_____ 8. Shortest portion of the male urethra   h. Myometrium

_____ 9. Transmits sperm to the ejaculatory duct   i. Suspensory ligament

FILL IN THE BLANKS

Fill in the blank spaces in the following sentences.

1. The thickened fold of mesentery that supports and stabilizes the position of each ovary is the

_____.

2. The _____ are fingerlike projections on the infundibulum that spread loosely over the surface of the ovaries.

3. The _____ are tightly coiled structures that store sperm for the final stages of maturation.

4. The _____ zone of the prostate surrounds the urethra.

5. The wall of the uterus is composed of three layers:

_____, _____,

and _____.

6. The _____ portion of the uterine tubes opens directly into the peritoneal cavity.

7. The _____ pouch is located between the uterus and rectum and is sometimes called the pouch of Douglas.

8. The muscle that originates from the ilium and sacrum and passes through the greater sciatic notch to insert on the greater trochanter is the

_____.

9. The pelvic brim is formed by the _____

line and the _____ line.

10. The upper portion of the acetabulum is created by the

_____.

SHORT ANSWER

1. Define the boundaries of the pelvic inlet and outlet.

2. Describe how the pelvic perineum is divided.

3. List the three gluteus muscles and define their combined function.

4. Describe the trigone of the bladder.

5. Describe the function of the fimbriae.

IDENTIFY

1. On Figure 8.7, coronal oblique CT of sacrum, label the following structures.

a. _____

b. _____

c. _____

d. _____

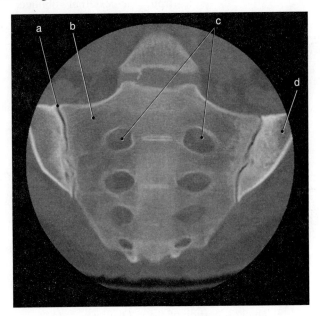

2. On Figure 8.29, axial MRI of pelvis, label the following structures.

a. _____

b. _____

c. _____

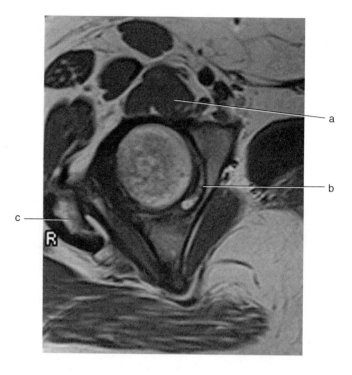

3. On Figure 8.3, coronal CT reformat of pelvis with acetabulum, label the following structures.

a. _____

b. _____

c. _____

d. _____

e. _____

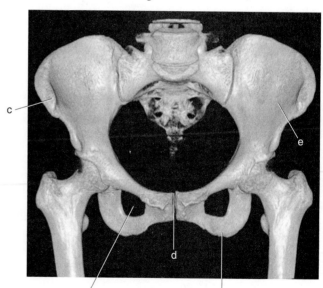

4. On Figure 8.27, axial MRI of pelvis, label the following structures.

a. _____

b. _____

c. _____

d. _____

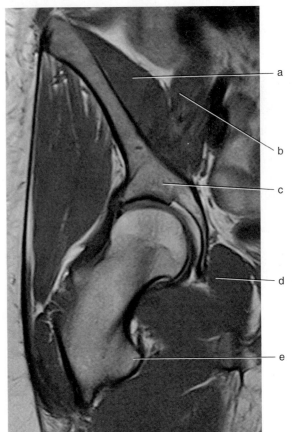

5. On Figure 8.13, coronal MRI of hip, label the following structures.

a. _____

b. _____

c. _____

d. _____

e. _____

6. On Figure 8.44, sagittal MRI of female pelvis, label the following structures.

a. _____

b. _____

c. _____

d. _____

e. _____

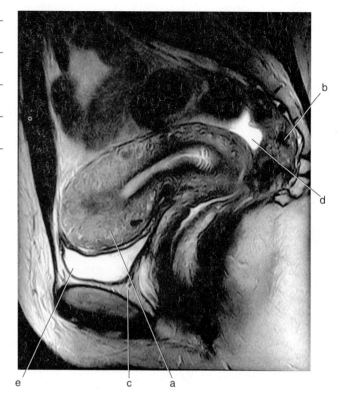

7. On Figure 8.63, axial CT of female pelvis, label the following structures.

a. _____

b. _____

c. _____

d. _____

e. _____

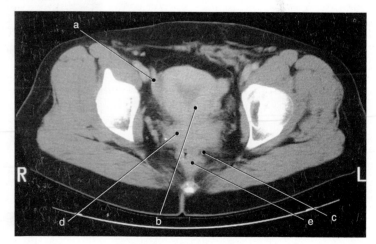

8. On Figure 8.70, axial MRI of female pelvis with ovaries, label the following structures.

a. _____

b. _____

c. _____

d. _____

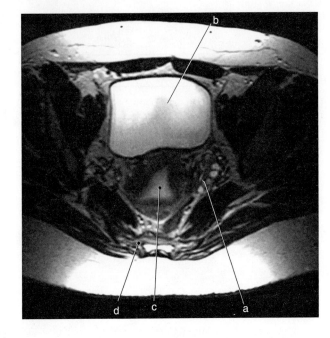

9. On Figure 8.95, axial CT of male pelvis, label the following structures.

a. _____

b. _____

c. _____

d. _____

e. _____

f. _____

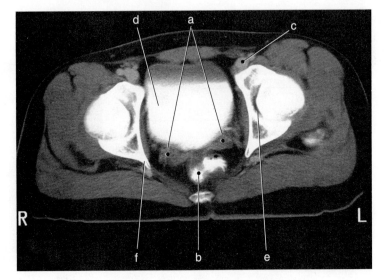

10. On Figure 8.96, sagittal MRI of male pelvis, label the following structures.

a. _____

b. _____

c. _____

d. _____

e. _____

f. _____

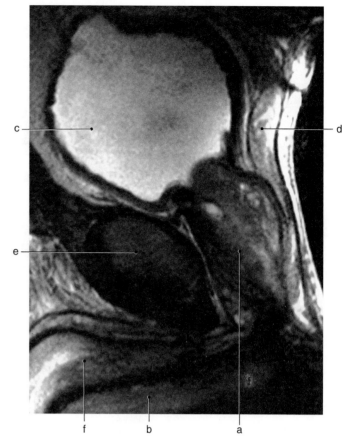

11. On Figure 8.28, axial CT of pelvis, label the following structures.

a. _____

b. _____

c. _____

d. _____

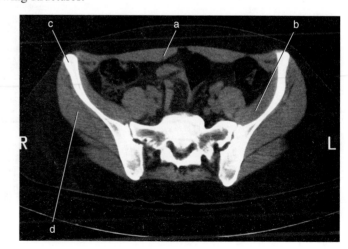

12. On Figure 8.24, coronal MRI of pelvis, label the following structures.

a. _____

b. _____

c. _____

d. _____

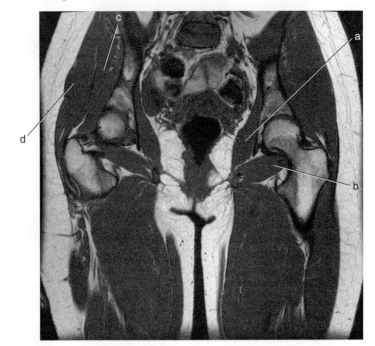

13. On Figure 8.34, axial MRI of male pelvis, label the following structures.

a. _____

b. _____

c. _____

d. _____

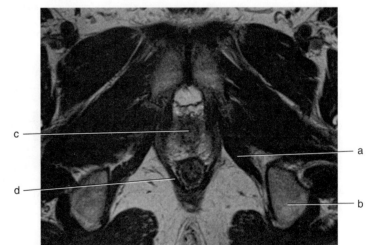

14. On Figure 8.47, coronal MRI of female pelvis, label the following structures.

a. _____

b. _____

c. _____

d. _____

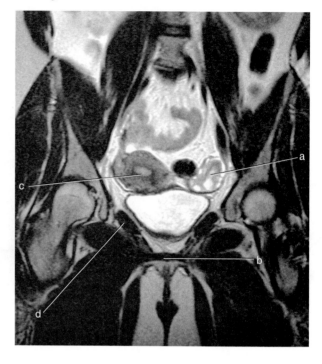

15. On Figure 8.90, axial MRI of male pelvis, label the following structures.

a. _____

b. _____

c. _____

d. _____

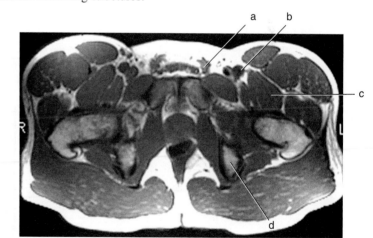

16. On Figure 8.82, coronal MRI of male pelvis, label the following structures.

a. _____

b. _____

c. _____

d. _____

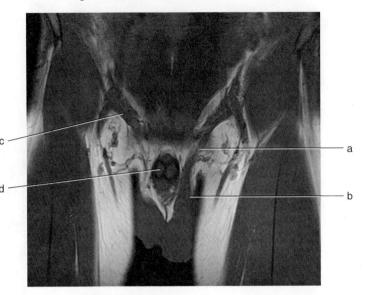

17. On Figure 8.118, 3D coronal CTA of iliac vessels, label the following structures.

a. _____

b. _____

c. _____

d. _____

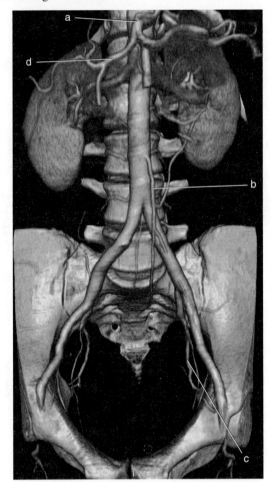

18. On Figure 8.6, coronal oblique MRI of sacrum, label the following structures.

a. _____

b. _____

c. _____

d. _____

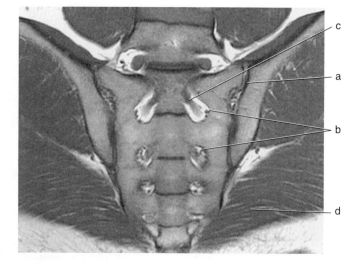

19. On Figure 8.19, 3D CT of pelvis, label the following structures.

a. _____

b. _____

c. _____

d. _____

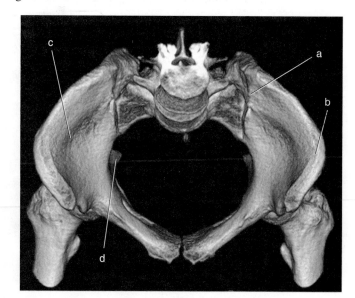

20. On Figure 8.32, axial MRI of male pelvis, label the following structures.

a. _____

b. _____

c. _____

d. _____

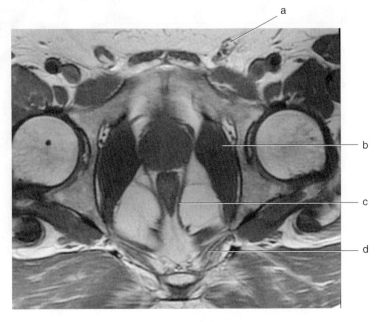

21. On Figure 8.46, sagittal MRI of male pelvis, label the following structures.

a. _____

b. _____

c. _____

d. _____

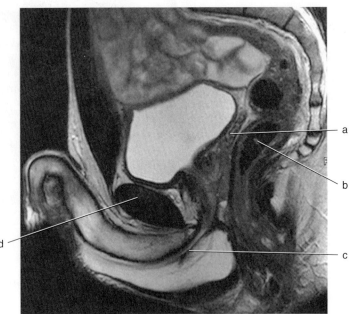

22. On Figure 8.53, axial CT of male pelvis, label the following structures.

a. _____

b. _____

c. _____

d. _____

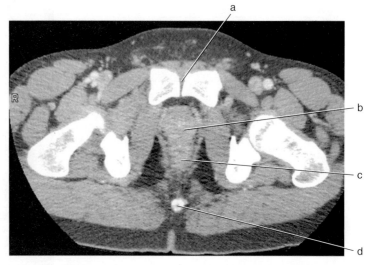

23. On Figure 8.69, coronal MRI of female pelvis, label the following structures.

a. _____

b. _____

c. _____

d. _____

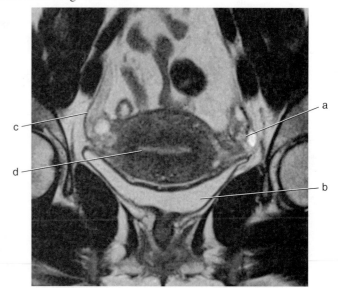

24. On Figure 8.73, coronal CT reformat of female pelvis, label the following structures.

a. _____

b. _____

c. _____

d. _____

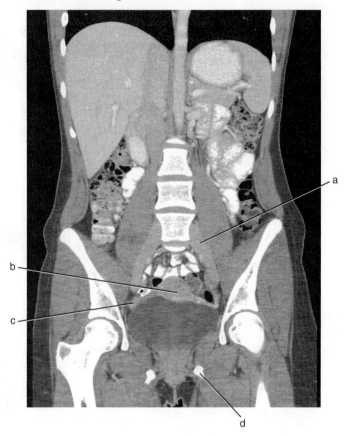

25. On Figure 8.99, axial MRI of male pelvis, label the following structures.

a. _____

b. _____

c. _____

d. _____

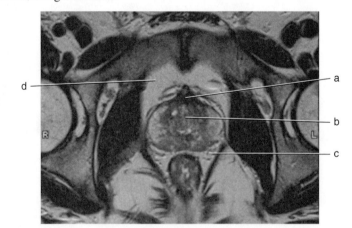

26. On Figure 8.104, axial MRI of male pelvis, label the following structures.

a. _____

b. _____

c. _____

d. _____

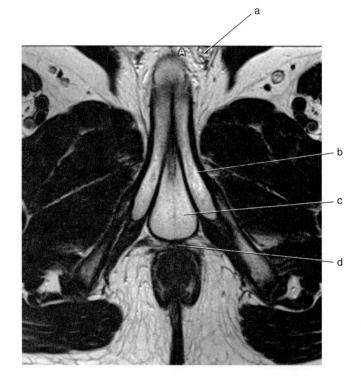

27. On Figure 8.125, axial MRI of hip, label the following structures.

a. _____

b. _____

c. _____

d. _____

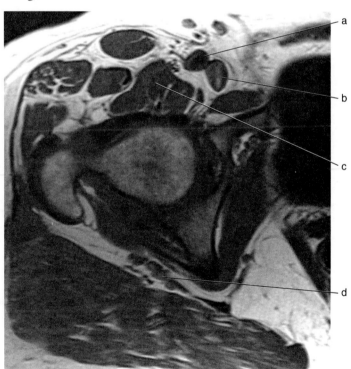

CASE STUDIES

Case Study 1

Cancer of the prostate gland is the second most common type of cancer in men, occurring with increasing frequency after the age of 55.

1. The glandular tissue of the prostate can be divided into zonal anatomy. What are the zones?

2. The ejaculatory ducts descend through the prostate in which zonal anatomy?

Case Study 2

A 42-year-old male complained of intermittent nausea, abdominal pain, and distension with standing. He was diagnosed with a bowel herniation through the inguinal canal (inguinal hernia).

1. Where is the inguinal canal located?

2. What structures normally pass through the inguinal canal?

9 Upper Extremity

OBJECTIVES

1. Identify the bony anatomy of the upper extremity.
2. Identify the components that contribute to the glenoid labrum.
3. Describe the joint capsules of the shoulder and elbow.
4. List and describe the ligaments and tendons of each upper extremity joint.
5. Identify and state the actions of the muscles as well as their origin and insertion sites.
6. Identify the major arteries and veins of the upper extremity.
7. List and identify the nerves that innervate the upper extremity.

After reading Chapter 9, see if you can complete the following problems.

MULTIPLE CHOICE

1. Which group of ligaments contributes to the formation of the glenoid labrum?
   a. Coracoclavicular
   b. Coracoacromial
   c. Glenoacromial
   d. Glenohumeral

2. Which rotator cuff muscle inserts on the lesser tubercle of the humerus?
   a. Supraspinatus
   b. Infraspinatus
   c. Subscapularis
   d. Teres minor

3. Which nerve is compressed in carpal tunnel syndrome?
   a. Ulnar
   b. Radial
   c. Median
   d. Thenar

4. What is the major stabilizing mechanism for the distal radioulnar joint?
   a. Carpal tunnel
   b. Triangular fibrocartilage
   c. Carpal bridge
   d. Flexor retinaculum

5. Which muscle is the main flexor of the forearm?
   a. Brachialis
   b. Triceps brachii
   c. Biceps brachii
   d. Pronator teres

6. Which rotator cuff muscle is located on the anterior surface of the scapula?
   a. Supraspinatus
   b. Infraspinatus
   c. Subscapularis
   d. Teres minor

7. Which rotator cuff tendon is the most frequently injured?
   a. Supraspinatus
   b. Infraspinatus
   c. Subscapularis
   d. Teres minor

8. The primary function of the glenoid labrum is to:
   a. Deepen the glenoid fossa
   b. Lubricate the joint capsule
   c. Serve as an attachment site for the rotator cuff muscles
   d. Protect the articular surface of the humeral head

9. Which ligament binds the radial head to the ulna?
   a. Anular
   b. Radial collateral
   c. Ulnar collateral
   d. Trochlear

10. What ligamentous structure spans the wrist to create an enclosure for the passage of tendons?
    a. Anular ligament
    b. Radial collateral ligament
    c. Flexor retinaculum
    d. Distal radioulnar tendon

11. Which of the following elbow joint ligaments consists of an anterior band, a posterior band, and a transverse band (ligament of Cooper)?
    a. Ulnar collateral
    b. Radial collateral
    c. Anular
    d. Quadrate

12. The most medial and superficial muscle located in the anterior compartment of the forearm is the:
    a. Pronator teres
    b. Flexor carpi ulnaris
    c. Digitorum profundus
    d. Pronator quadratus

13. Which of the following finger ligaments prevents separation of the metacarpals?
    a. Accessory collateral
    b. Palmar
    c. Collateral
    d. Deep transverse metacarpal

14. Which of the following arteries courses inferiorly on the medial side of the humerus then continues anterior to the cubital fossa of the elbow and is the principal arterial supply to the arm?
    a. Axillary
    b. Brachial
    c. Radial
    d. Ulnar

15. The cephalic vein continues superiorly as which vein?
    a. Basilic
    b. Subclavian
    c. Axillary
    d. Radial

TRUE/FALSE

Circle either True or False for each of the following statements.

True/False 1. The supraspinatus tendon inserts on lesser tubercle of the humerus.

True/False 2. The trochlea of the humerus articulates with the capitellum of the radius.

True/False 3. The pronator teres muscle has two heads of origin.

True/False 4. The ulnar nerve is located between the medial epicondyle of the humerus and the olecranon process.

True/False 5. In the middle of the body of the humerus, on the anterior surface, is a roughened area called the deltoid tuberosity.

True/False 6. The subscapular bursa is the main bursa of the shoulder joint.

True/False 7. The radial tuberosity serves as the attachment point for the biceps brachii muscle.

True/False 8. All five of the superficial muscles in the ventral group of the forearm have an origin from the common flexor tendon.

True/False 9. The common interosseous artery begins at the level of the radial head and courses beneath the brachioradialis muscle.

True/False 10. The brachial veins begin in the elbow from the union of the ulnar and radial veins and end in the axillary vein.

FILL IN THE BLANKS

Fill in the blank spaces in the following sentences.

1. Located on the anterior surface of the scapula is a beaklike process termed the _____.

2. The _____ tendon blends with the superior glenoid labrum.

3. A large depression located on the anterior surface of the distal humerus is termed the _____.

4. The _____ ligament reinforces the medial side of the elbow.

5. The _____ is an extensor muscle of the lateral forearm, attaching to the radial styloid process.

6. The extension of the axillary artery that descends along the anterior aspect of the arm is termed the

   _____.

7. A ligamentous structure known as the _____

   _____ creates an enclosure across the carpal tunnel for the passage of tendons and the median nerve.

8. The _____ group of tendons collectively flexes the fingers and wrist.

Write in an answer next to the "x" in the following tables.

Muscles Connecting the Upper Extremity to the Vertebral Column (see Table 9.1)

Muscle	Origin	Insertion	Primary Actions
x _____	External occipital protuberance, ligamentum nuchae, spinous processes of C7-T12	Clavicle, acromion, and spine of the scapula	Stabilize, elevate, retract, and depress scapula
Levator scapula	Transverse processes of C1-C4	x _____	x _____
x _____	Spinous process of T6-T12, iliac crest, and inferior 3-4 ribs	Intertubercular groove of the humerus	Extend, medially rotate, and adduct the humerus
Rhomboid major	Ligamentum nuchae and spinous processes of C7-T1	x _____	x _____
Rhomboid minor	x _____	Medial border of scapula	Retracts scapula and fixes scapula to thoracic wall

Scapular Muscles (see Table 9.2)

Muscle	Proximal/Medial Attachment	Distal/Lateral Attachment	Primary Action
Deltoid	Clavicle, acromion, and spine of scapula	x _____	x _____
x _____	Inferior angle of scapula	Intertubercular groove of humerus	Adducts and medially rotates humerus
Teres minor	x _____	Greater tubercle of humerus	x _____
x _____	Supraspinous fossa of scapula	Greater tubercle of humerus	Abducts humerus and stabilizes glenohumeral joint
Infraspinatus	x _____	Greater tubercle of humerus	x _____
Subscapularis	Subscapular fossa of scapula	x _____	Medially rotates humerus and stabilizes glenohumeral joint

Muscles Connecting the Upper Extremity to the Anterior and Lateral Thoracic Wall (see Table 9.3)

Muscle	Proximal/Medial Attachment	Distal/Lateral Attachment	Primary Action
x _____	Medial half of clavicle, manubrium and body of sternum, and six upper costal cartilages	Lateral lip intertubercular groove of humerus	Adducts, medially rotates, and flexes humerus
Pectoralis minor	Anterior surface of ribs 3-5	x _____	Depresses and downwardly rotates scapula, assists in scapular protraction, and stabilizes scapula
Serratus anterior	x _____	Medial border of scapula	Rotates, stabilizes, and protracts scapula
Subclavius	First rib and cartilage	x _____	x _____

Muscles of the Upper Arm (see Table 9.4)

Muscle	Proximal Attachment	Distal Attachment	Primary Action
Biceps brachii	Long head—supraglenoid tubercle of scapula Short head—coracoid process of scapula	x _____	x _____
Brachialis	x _____	Ulnar tuberosity and coronoid process	x _____
x _____	Coracoid process of scapula	Middle third medial surface of humerus	Assists to flex and adduct the arm
Triceps brachii	Long head—infraglenoid tubercle of scapula Medial head—posterior surface of humerus below the radial groove Lateral head—posterior surface of humerus below greater tubercle	x _____	Chief extensor of forearm, long head steadies head of humerus if abducted
Anconeus	Lateral epicondyle of humerus	x _____	Assists triceps brachii in extension of elbow

1. What is the triangular fibrocartilage complex (TFCC)?

2. What is the glenoid labrum, and which ligaments contribute to its formation?

3. What is the anular ligament?

4. List the four projections of the scapula.

5. The supraglenoid tubercle and infraglenoid tubercle of the scapula serve as attachment sites for which muscles?

6. Describe the articular joint capsule of the shoulder joint.

7. List the function of the intercarpal (intrinsic) ligaments of the wrist.

8. Describe the flexor retinaculum.

9. List the functions of the palmar and dorsal tendon groups.

10. List the nerves that supply the muscles of the forearm and hand.

IDENTIFY

1. On Figure 9.18, coronal oblique MRI of shoulder, label the following structures.

    a. _____

    b. _____

    c. _____

    d. _____

    e. _____

    f. _____

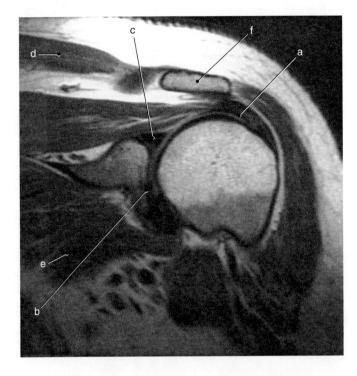

2. On Figure 9.15, axial CT of shoulder, midjoint, label the following structures.

a. _____

b. _____

c. _____

d. _____

e. _____

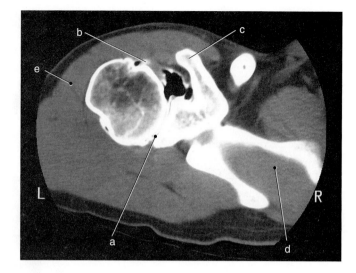

3. On Figure 9.10, sagittal oblique MRI of shoulder, label the following structures.

a. _____

b. _____

c. _____

d. _____

e. _____

f. _____

g. _____

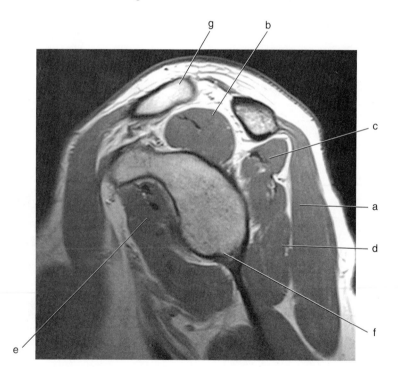

4. On Figure 9.76, coronal MRI of elbow, label the following structures.

a. _____

b. _____

c. _____

d. _____

e. _____

f. _____

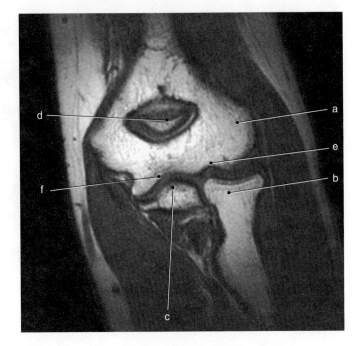

5. On Figure 9.91, axial MRI of elbow, label the following structures.

a. _____

b. _____

c. _____

d. _____

e. _____

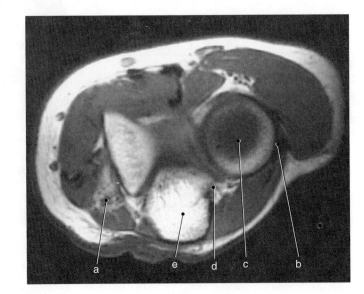

6. On Figure 9.80, sagittal MRI of elbow, label the following structures.

a. _____

b. _____

c. _____

d. _____

e. _____

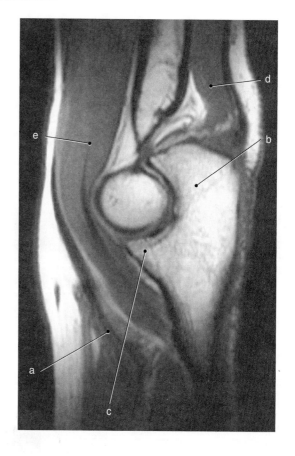

7. On Figure 9.100, axial CT of forearm muscles, label the following structures.

a. _____

b. _____

c. _____

d. _____

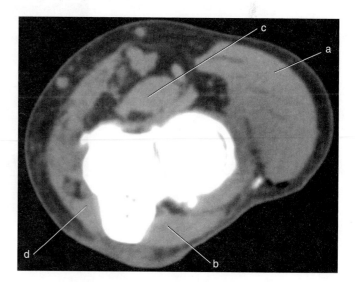

8. On Figure 9.119, coronal CT reformat of wrist, label the following structures.

a. _____

b. _____

c. _____

d. _____

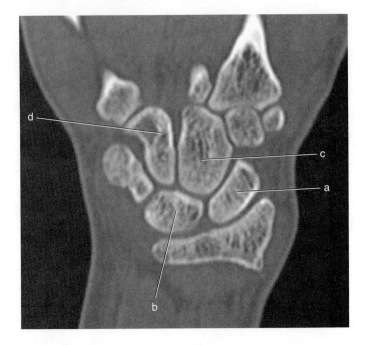

9. On Figure 9.131, axial MRI of wrist, label the following structures.

a. _____

b. _____

c. _____

d. _____

e. _____

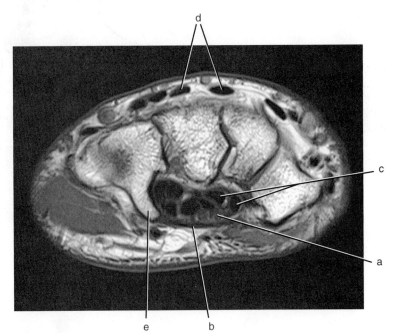

10. On Figure 9.9, 3D CT of superior aspect of scapula, label the following structures.

a. _____

b. _____

c. _____

d. _____

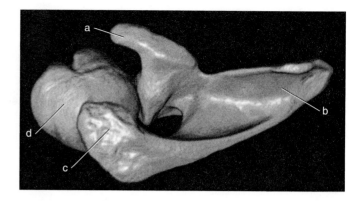

11. On Figure 9.14, axial MRI of shoulder, label the following structures.

a. _____

b. _____

c. _____

d. _____

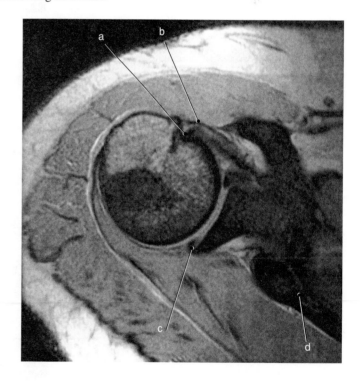

12. On Figure 9.22, sagittal oblique MRI of shoulder, label the following structures.

a. _____

b. _____

c. _____

d. _____

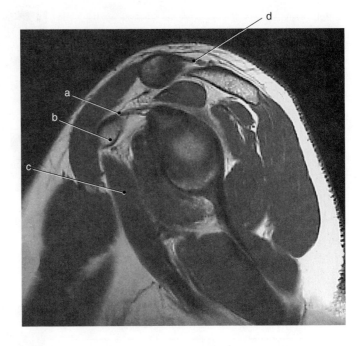

13. On Figure 9.32, axial MRI of shoulder, post-arthrogram label the following structures.

a. _____

b. _____

c. _____

d. _____

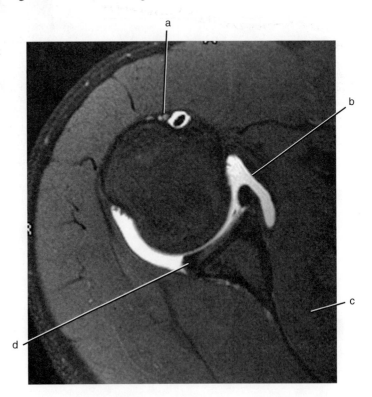

14. On Figure 9.97, axial MRI of forearm muscles, label the following structures.

a. _____

b. _____

c. _____

d. _____

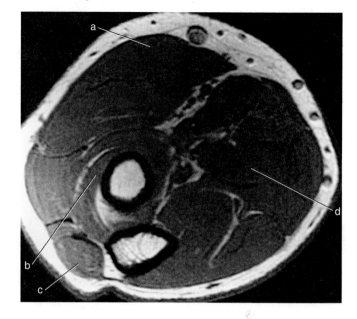

15. On Figure 9.105, sagittal MRI of forearm muscles, label the following structures.

a. _____

b. _____

c. _____

d. _____

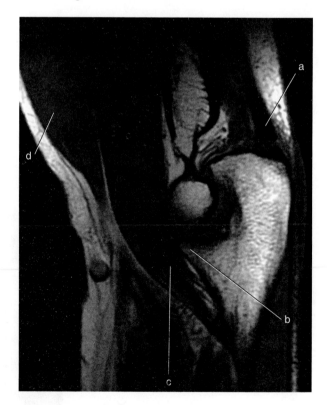

16. On Figure 9.145, sagittal MRI of wrist, label the following structures.

a. _____

b. _____

c. _____

d. _____

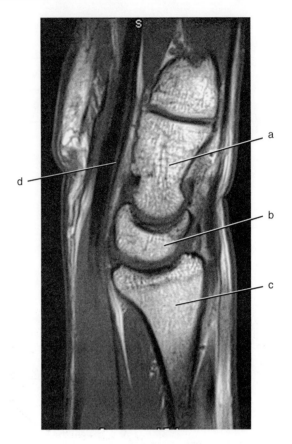

17. On Figure 9.130, axial MRI of wrist, label the following structures.

a. _____

b. _____

c. _____

d. _____

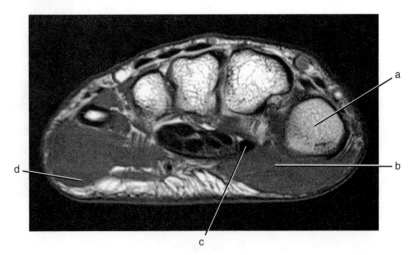

18. On Figure 9.151, axial MRI of hand, label the following structures.

a. _____

b. _____

c. _____

d. _____

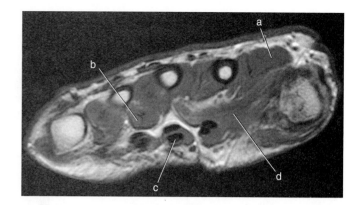

19. On Figure 9.6, coronal oblique MRI of shoulder, label the following structures.

a. _____

b. _____

c. _____

d. _____

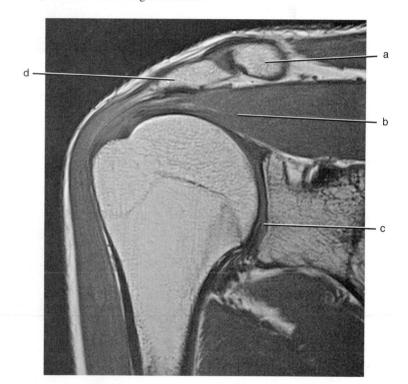

20. On Figure 9.27, axial MRI of shoulder, label the following structures.

a. _____

b. _____

c. _____

d. _____

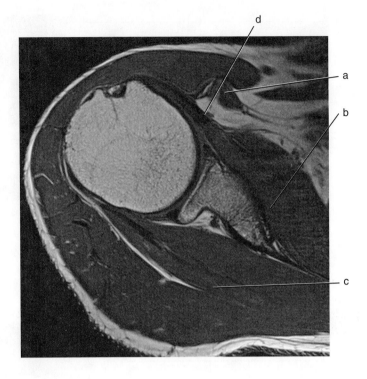

21. On Figure 9.28, coronal oblique MRI of shoulder, post-arthrogram, label the following structures.

a. _____

b. _____

c. _____

d. _____

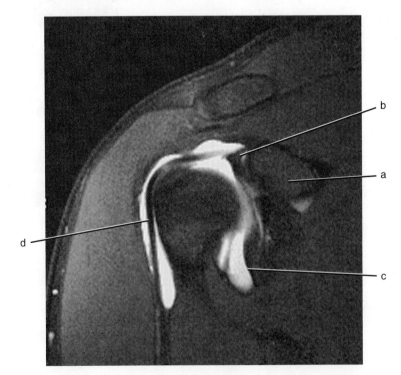

22. On Figure 9.31, axial MRI of shoulder, post-arthrogram, label the following structures.

a. _____

b. _____

c. _____

d. _____

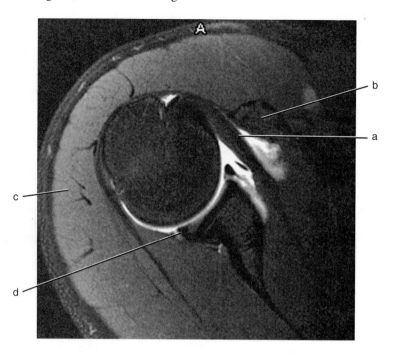

23. On Figure 9.66, axial MRI of midhumerus, arm, label the following structures.

a. _____

b. _____

c. _____

d. _____

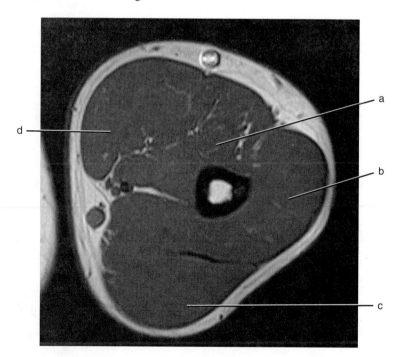

24. On Figure 9.113, 3D CT of carpal tunnel, label the following structures.

a. _____

b. _____

c. _____

d. _____

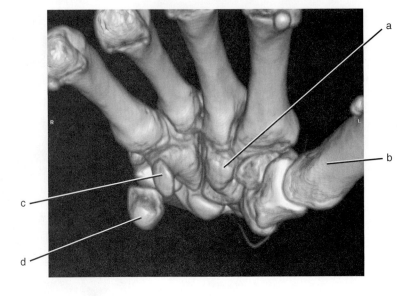

25. On Figure 9.125, coronal MRI of wrist, label the following structures.

a. _____

b. _____

c. _____

d. _____

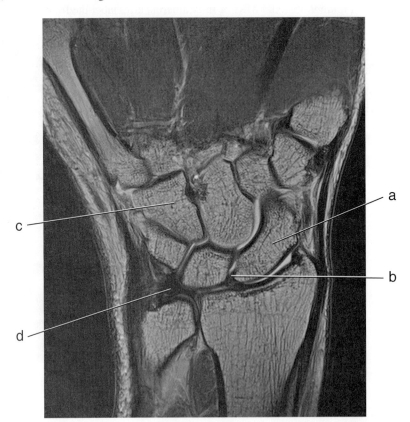

26. On Figure 9.133, axial MRI of wrist, label the following structures.

a. _____

b. _____

c. _____

d. _____

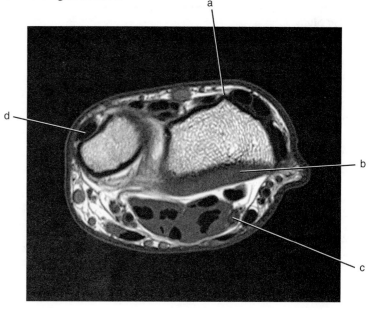

Case Study 1

A 16-year-old male was playing basketball and fell on his outstretched hand. Over the next 2 weeks he complained of ulnar-sided wrist pain and grinding within the joint, along with a limited range of motion. He was diagnosed with a triangular fibrocartilage complex (TFCC) tear.

1. Where is the TFCC located?

2. What is the function of the TFCC?

Case Study 2

Adhesive capsulitis or frozen shoulder is a condition that occurs when the joint capsule thickens and tightens around the shoulder joint, limiting its range of motion.

1. What muscles and ligaments strengthen the joint capsule of the shoulder?

2. What are two openings located in the joint capsule of the shoulder?

10 Lower Extremity

OBJECTIVES

1. Identify the bony anatomy of the lower extremity.
2. Identify and state the actions of the lower extremity muscles as well as their origins and insertions.
3. Describe the labrum and articular capsule of the hip.
4. List and describe the ligaments, retinacula, and tendons of the lower extremity joints.
5. Define and identify the meniscus and articular capsule of the knee.
6. Identify the bursae of the hip and knee.
7. List and identify the major arteries and veins of the lower extremity.
8. Describe the nerves that innervate the lower extremity.

After reading Chapter 10, see if you can complete the following problems.

MULTIPLE CHOICE

1. What structure deepens the acetabulum to increase stability of the hip joint?
   a. Articular cartilage
   b. Fovea capitis
   c. Acetabular labrum
   d. Obturator internus muscle

2. What structure contains the artery to the femoral head?
   a. Ligamentum teres
   b. Acetabular labrum
   c. Greater trochanter
   d. Transverse ligament

3. What is the largest peripheral nerve in the body?
   a. Femoral
   b. Sacral
   c. Sciatic
   d. Iliac

4. What is the strongest ligament in the ankle?
   a. Spring
   b. Deltoid
   c. Lateral
   d. Interosseous

5. What structure cushions the articulation between the femoral condyles and the tibial plateaus?
   a. Popliteal bursae
   b. Menisci
   c. Patellar ligaments
   d. Cruciate ligaments

6. Which ligament in the ankle helps to maintain the longitudinal arch of the foot?
   a. Spring
   b. Deltoid
   c. Lateral
   d. Interosseous

7. What structure provides weight-bearing support to the medial side of the ankle?
   a. Posterior facet
   b. Sinus tarsi
   c. Sustentaculum tali
   d. Navicular

8. What group of tendons in the ankle does the extensor hallucis longus belong to?
   a. Posterior
   b. Anterior
   c. Medial
   d. Lateral

9. What group of muscles act to flex the hip joint and extend the knee?
   a. Anterior
   b. Posterior
   c. Medial
   d. Lateral

10. What tendon is an extension of the gastrocnemius muscle?
    a. Tibialis anterior
    b. Extensor digitorum longus
    c. Peroneus longus
    d. Achilles

11. Which muscles act as plantar flexors, but also stabilize the lateral ankle and longitudinal arch of the foot?
    a. Peroneus
    b. Tibialis anterior
    c. Gastrocnemius
    d. Plantaris

12. Which muscle (or muscles) is a prominent flexor of the foot and is responsible for giving the calf its shape on the back of the leg?
    a. Peroneus
    b. Tibialis anterior
    c. Gastrocnemius
    d. Plantaris

13. Which of the following ligaments provide medial support to the ankle joint?
    a. Spring
    b. Interosseous
    c. Deltoid
    d. Plantar

14. The femoral artery is an extension of which artery?
    a. Internal iliac
    b. External iliac
    c. Medial circumflex femoral
    d. Lateral circumflex femoral

15. The great saphenous vein ascends the medial aspect of the leg and thigh to drain into which vein?
    a. Small saphenous
    b. Femoral
    c. External iliac
    d. Internal iliac

TRUE/FALSE

Circle either True or False for each of the following statements.

True/False   1. The transverse acetabular ligament creates a fibrocartilaginous rim attached to the margin of the acetabulum that deepens the fossa.

True/False   2. The patellar ligament is an extension of the quadriceps tendon.

True/False   3. The great saphenous vein ascends the lateral surface of the leg.

True/False   4. The tarsal canal widens laterally to form the sustentaculum tali.

True/False   5. The gastrocnemius muscle is a prominent flexor of the leg. It consists of two heads arising from the femoral condyles and inserts on the calcaneus via the Achilles tendon.

True/False   6. The femoral head is covered entirely by articular cartilage, with the exception of a small centrally located pit termed the fovea centralis.

True/False   7. The lesser trochanter of the femur is the insertion site for the tendon of the iliopsoas major muscle.

True/False   8. The two gemellus muscles are located along the superior and inferior boundaries of the obturator internus muscle and tendon.

True/False   9. A small projection located above the medial epicondyle of the femur is termed the adductor tubercle.

True/False   10. The oblique and arcuate popliteal ligaments help reinforce the ventral surface of the knee joint capsule.

FILL IN THE BLANKS

1. The _____ of the hip forms a sleeve that encloses the hip joint and most of the femoral neck.

2. The posterior surface of the tibia has an obliquely oriented bony ridge termed the _____.

3. The menisci cushion the articulation between the femoral condyles and the tibial plateaus and are commonly divided into the _____ and _____ horns.

4. The _____ bursa is a large extension of the synovial capsule located between the femur and quadriceps tendon.

5. On the medial surface of the calcaneus is a shelflike process termed the _____.

6. The _____ is a canal that contains blood vessels, fat, and the cervical ligament and widens laterally to form the sinus tarsi.

7. The _____ is approximately 80 layers thick, creating some of the thickest fascia within the human body.

8. The femoral nerve terminates at the _____ to innervate the skin on the medial side of the leg and foot.

9. From the lateral side of the foot, the _____ vein passes posterolaterally to join the popliteal vein.

10. The muscles of the foot are divided into the muscles of the _____ and _____ of the foot.

Write in an answer next to the "x" in the following table.

Muscles of the Gluteal Region

Muscle	Proximal Insertion	Distal Insertion	Action
x _____	Ilium, sacrum, coccyx	Gluteal tuberosity of greater trochanter	Extensor of the hip, maintains erect position of the body
Gluteus medius	Iliac crest	Greater trochanter	Abducts and medially rotates the thigh
Gluteus minimus	Gluteal surface of ilium	x _____	Abducts and medially rotates the thigh
x _____	Sacrum	Greater trochanter	Lateral rotation and abduction of the thigh
Obturator internus	Obturator foramen	Greater trochanter	Lateral rotation and abduction of the thigh
Obturator externus	Obturator foramen	Greater trochanter	Lateral rotation of the thigh
Superior gemellus	x _____	Greater trochanter	Lateral rotation and abduction of the thigh
Inferior gemellus	Ischial tuberosity	Greater trochanter	Lateral rotation and abduction of the thigh
Quadratus femoris	Ischial tuberosity	Intertrochanteric crest	Lateral rotation of the thigh

SHORT ANSWER

1. Describe the iliotibial (IT) band.

2. List the muscles of the medial thigh compartment and their collective function.

3. List the muscles that are collectively known as the hamstrings.

4. List the three articulations of the subtalar joint.

5. Describe the retinacula in the ankle.

IDENTIFY

1. On Figure 10.3, axial CT of hip joint, post-arthrogram label the following structures.

   a. _____

   b. _____

   c. _____

   d. _____

   e. _____

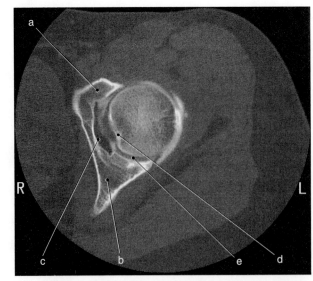

2. On Figure 10.4, axial MRI of hip, label the following structures.

a. _____

b. _____

c. _____

d. _____

e. _____

f. _____

g. _____

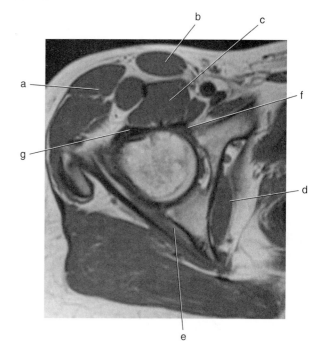

3. On Figure 10.6, coronal MRI of hip, label the following structures.

a. _____

b. _____

c. _____

d. _____

e. _____

f. _____

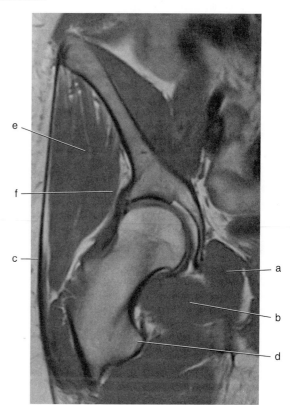

4. On Figure 10.59, coronal MRI of knee, label the following structures.

a. _____

b. _____

c. _____

d. _____

e. _____

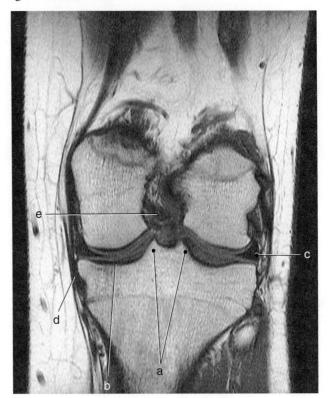

5. On Figure 10.88, sagittal MRI of knee, label the following structures.

a. _____

b. _____

c. _____

d. _____

e. _____

f. _____

g. _____

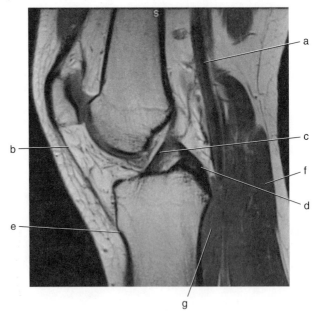

6. On Figure 10.130, axial CT of ankle and foot, label the following structures.

a. _____

b. _____

c. _____

d. _____

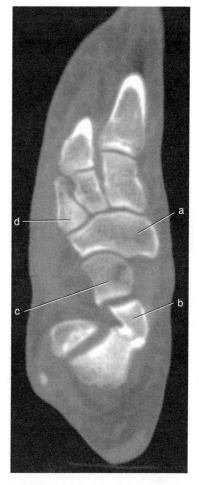

7. On Figure 10.122, sagittal MRI of calcaneus, label the following structures.

a. _____

b. _____

c. _____

d. _____

e. _____

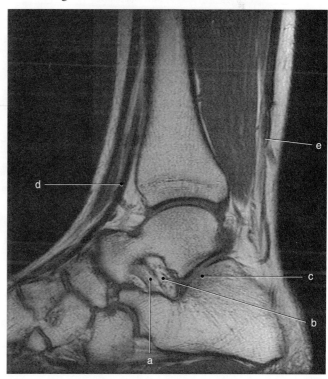

8. On Figure 10.127, axial MRI of ankle, label the following structures.

a. _____

b. _____

c. _____

d. _____

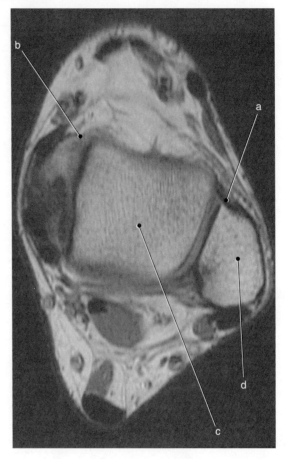

9. On Figure 10.30, sagittal MRI of hip with muscles, label the following structures.

a. _____

b. _____

c. _____

d. _____

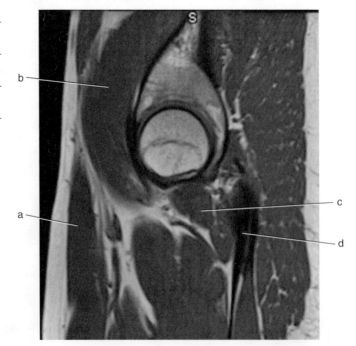

10. On Figure 10.45, axial MRI of midfemur, label the following structures.

    a. _____

    b. _____

    c. _____

    d. _____

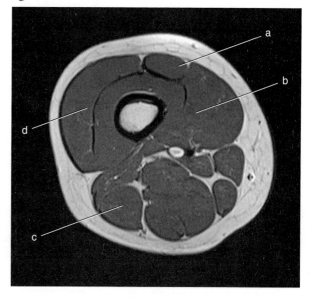

11. On Figure 10.49, coronal MRI of hip and thigh muscles, label the following structures.

    a. _____

    b. _____

    c. _____

    d. _____

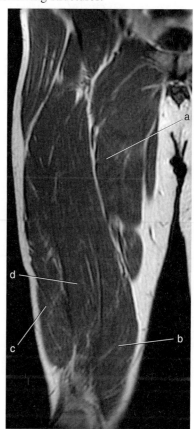

12. On Figure 10.75, coronal MRI of knee, label the following structures.

   a. _____

   b. _____

   c. _____

   d. _____

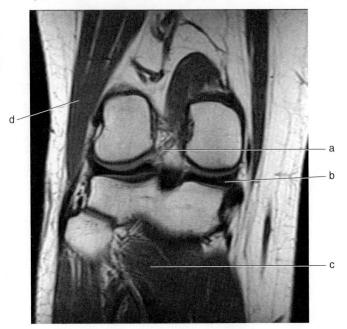

13. On Figure 10.97, axial CT of knee, label the following structures.

   a. _____

   b. _____

   c. _____

   d. _____

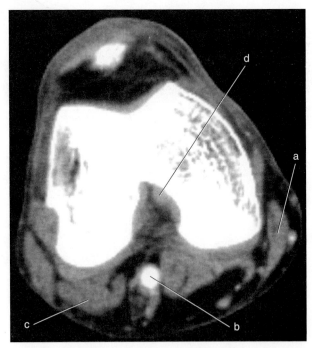

14. On Figure 10.107, axial MRI of proximal lower leg, label the following structures.

a. _____

b. _____

c. _____

d. _____

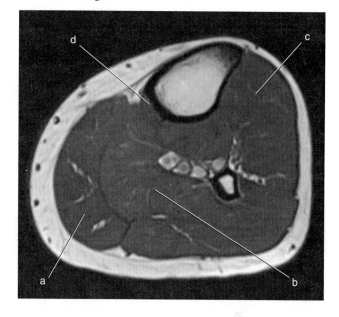

15. On Figure 10.109, axial MRI of distal lower leg, label the following structures.

a. _____

b. _____

c. _____

d. _____

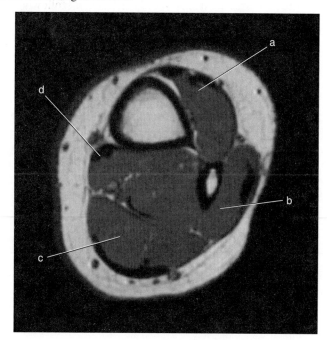

16. On Figure 10.112, sagittal MRI scan of lower leg, label the following structures.

a. _____

b. _____

c. _____

d. _____

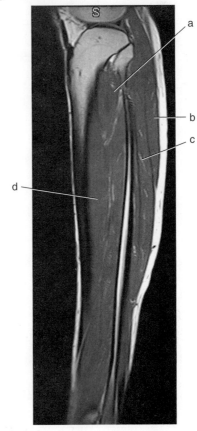

17. On Figure 10.149, axial MRI of foot, label the following structures.

a. _____

b. _____

c. _____

d. _____

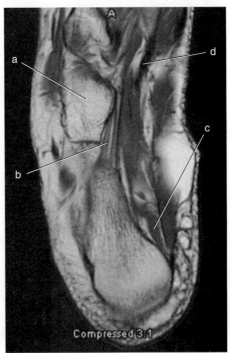

18. On Figure 10.157, coronal MRI of ankle ligaments and tendons, label the following structures.

a. _____

b. _____

c. _____

d. _____

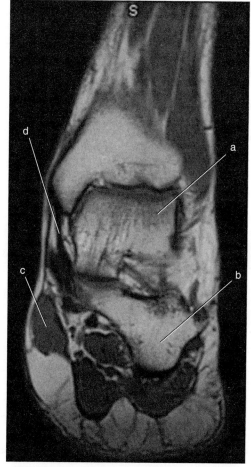

19. On Figure 10.158, coronal MRI of ankle ligaments and tendons, label the following structures.

a. _____

b. _____

c. _____

d. _____

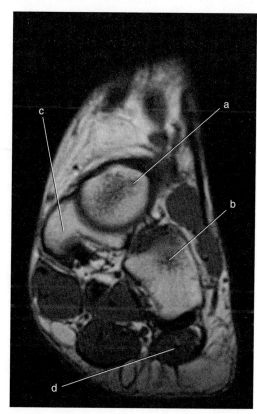

20. On Figure 10.159, coronal MRI of ankle ligaments and tendons, label the following structures.

a. _____

b. _____

c. _____

d. _____

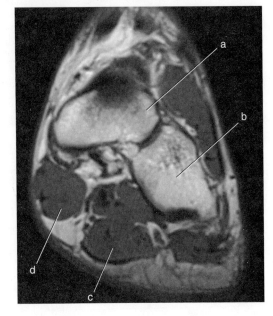

21. On Figure 10.169, 3D CTA of lower extremities, label the following structures.

a. _____

b. _____

c. _____

d. _____

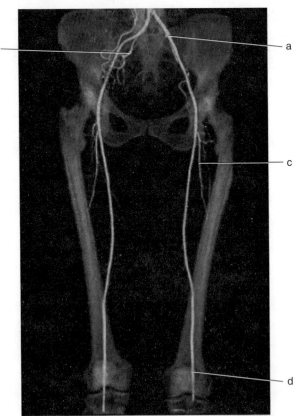

22. On Figure 10.22, axial oblique MRI, post-arthrogram, of hip, label the following structures.

a. _____

b. _____

c. _____

d. _____

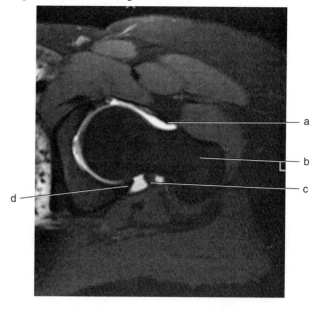

23. On Figure 10.24, coronal MRI, post-arthrogram, of hip, label the following structures.

a. _____

b. _____

c. _____

d. _____

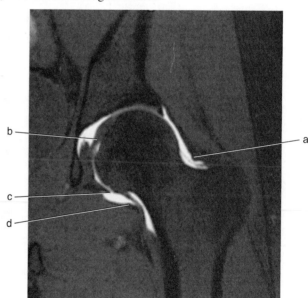

24. On Figure 10.45, axial MRI of distal femur, label the following structures.

a. _____

b. _____

c. _____

d. _____

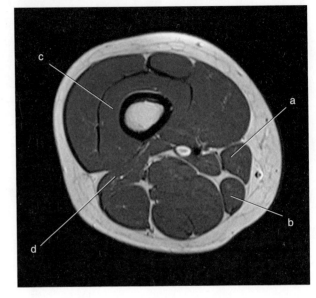

25. On Figure 10.57, axial MRI of right knee, label the following structures.

a. _____

b. _____

c. _____

d. _____

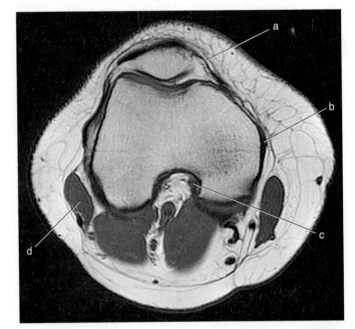

26. On Figure 10.64, axial MRI of knee with tibiofibular articulation, label the following structures.

a. _____

b. _____

c. _____

d. _____

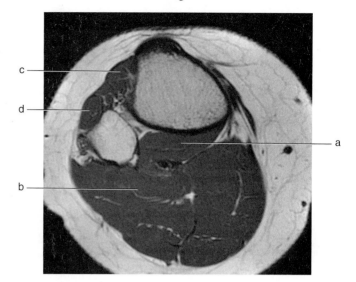

27. On Figure 10.67, axial MRI of ankle with malleoli, label the following structures.

a. _____

b. _____

c. _____

d. _____

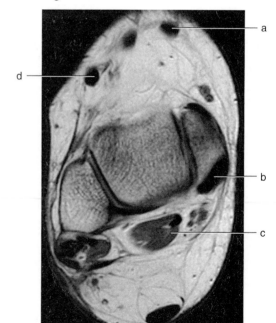

181

28. On Figure 10.87, sagittal MRI of knee, label the following structures.

a. _____

b. _____

c. _____

d. _____

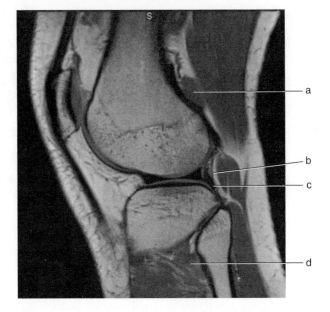

29. On Figure 10.96, axial MRI of knee, label the following structures.

a. _____

b. _____

c. _____

d. _____

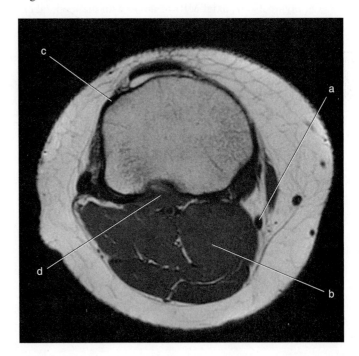

30. On Figure 10.118c, 3D CT of foot, lateral view, label the following structures.

a. _____

b. _____

c. _____

d. _____

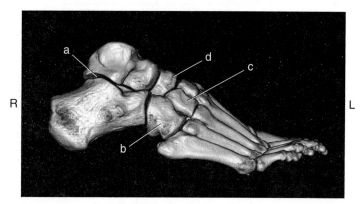

31. On Figure 10.144, axial MRI of ankle, label the following structures.

a. _____

b. _____

c. _____

d. _____

e. _____

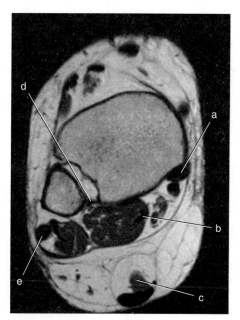

32. On Figure 10.162, coronal MRI of metatarsals, label the following structures.

a. _____

b. _____

c. _____

d. _____

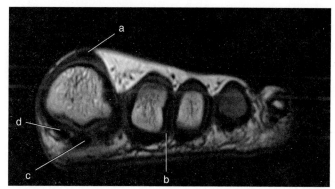

CASE STUDIES

Case Study 1

A 17-year-old male soccer player experienced tingling and burning along the medial side of the ankle and along the bottom of the foot. After a clinical examination and electrodiagnostic studies were completed, the patient was diagnosed with tarsal tunnel syndrome.

1. What is the tarsal tunnel?

2. What structures pass through the tarsal tunnel?

Case Study 2

A 14-year-old female was playing soccer when she heard an audible pop and felt her knee lock up. She complained of severe pain, and her knee swelled significantly. An MRI confirmed that she had a large meniscal tear that would require arthoscopic surgery for repair.

1. Which meniscus is most mobile?

2. What structures arise from the posterior horn of the lateral meniscus?

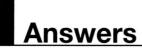

Answers

CHAPTER 1: INTRODUCTION TO SECTIONAL ANATOMY

MATCHING

Directional Terminology

1. d	11. c
2. k	12. r
3. e	13. p
4. l	14. a
5. n	15. h
6. f	16. i
7. q	17. j
8. m	18. s
9. b	19. g
10. o	

Regional Terminology

1. e	7. d
2. l	8. i
3. f	9. a
4. b	10. h
5. c	11. k
6. j	12. g

FILL IN THE TABLE

Internal Landmarks

Landmark	Location
Aortic arch	2.5 cm below jugular notch
Aortic bifurcation	L4-L5
Carina	T4-T5, sternal angle
Carotid bifurcation	Upper border of thyroid cartilage
Celiac trunk	4 cm above transpyloric plane
Circle of Willis	Suprasellar cistern
Common iliac vein bifurcation	Upper margin of sacroiliac joint
Conus medullaris	T12 to L1, L2
Heart: apex	Fifth intercostal space, left midclavicular line
Heart: base	Level of second and third costal cartilages behind sternum
Inferior mesenteric artery	4 cm above bifurcation of abdominal aorta
Portal vein	Posterior to pancreatic neck

Landmark	Location
Renal arteries	Anterior to L1, inferior to superior mesenteric artery
Superior mesenteric artery	2 cm above transpyloric plane
Thyroid gland	Thyroid cartilage
Vocal cords	Midway between superior and inferior border of thyroid cartilage

SHORT ANSWER

1. Sagittal—a vertical plane that passes through the body, dividing it into right and left portions
Coronal—a vertical plane that passes through the body, dividing it into anterior and posterior portions
Axial—a horizontal plane that passes through the body, dividing it into superior and inferior portions
Oblique—a plane that passes diagonally between the axes of two other planes
2. The two main body cavities are the dorsal and ventral cavities. The dorsal cavity includes the cranial and spinal cavities, and the ventral cavity is subdivided into the thoracic and abdominopelvic cavities.
3. Any three of the following: right lobe of the liver, gallbladder, right kidney, portions of the stomach, small, and large intestines
4. Any six of the following: right hypochondrium, epigastrium, left hypochondrium, right lateral, umbilical, left lateral, right inguinal, hypogastrium, left inguinal
5. It represents the attenuating properties or density of each tissue.
6. Any CT number above zero will represent tissue denser than water and will appear in progressively lighter shades of gray to white.
7. In MR, the gray scale represents the specific tissue relaxation properties of T1, T2, and proton density.
8. A ray from the camera's viewpoint is directed to stop at the maximum voxel value. With this method, only the brightest voxels will be mapped into the final image.
9. In volume rendering, the contributions of each voxel are summed along the course of the ray from the camera's viewpoint. The process is repeated numerous times to determine each pixel value that will be displayed in the final image.
10. The two commonly used horizontal planes are the transpyloric and transtubercular planes, and the two sagittal planes are the two midclavicular.

CHAPTER 2: CRANIUM AND FACIAL BONES

Matching

1. f   4. b
2. d   5. a
3. c   6. e

TRUE/FALSE

1. False—The largest immovable facial bone is the maxilla.
2. True
3. False—The maxillary sinuses drain into the middle nasal meatus.
4. False—The sphenoid sinuses are typically paired and separated by a septum.
5. True
6. True
7. False—The vestibule is a part of the inner ear, but it is involved with balance and equilibrium.
8. False—The bony orbit is composed of the frontal, sphenoid, and ethmoid bones of the cranium and the lacrimal, palatine, maxillary, and zygoma of the facial bones.
9. False—The lacrimal gland is located in the superior lateral portion of the orbit.
10. True

FILL IN THE BLANKS

1. Round window
2. Foramen magnum
3. Clivus
4. Temporal
5. Sphenoid
6. Masseter
7. Vomer
8. Articular eminence
9. Cribriform plate
10. Tuberculum sellae
11. Ethmoid bulla
12. Rotundum, ovale, and spinosum
13. Collateral ligaments

FILL IN THE TABLE (see Table 2.3)

Paranasal sinus drainage location

Sinus	Drainage Location
Ethmoid: anterior	Middle nasal meatus
Ethmoid: posterior	Superior nasal meatus
Maxillary	Middle nasal meatus
Sphenoid	Sphenoethmoidal recess
Frontal	Middle nasal meatus

Foramina and Fissures of the Skull (see Table 2.2)

Bone	Foramen/Fissure	Major Structures Using Passageway
Frontal	Supraorbital foramen (or notch) Frontal foramen (or notch)	Supraorbital nerve and artery Frontal artery and nerve
Ethmoid	Cribriform plate	Olfactory nerve (I)
Sphenoid	Foramen rotundum Foramen ovale Foramen spinosum Pterygoid canal Optic canal Superior orbital fissure	Maxillary branch of trigeminal nerve (V) Mandibular branch of trigeminal nerve (V) Middle meningeal artery Petrosal nerve Optic nerve and ophthalmic artery Ophthalmic vein, Oculomotor nerve (III), trochlear nerve (IV), ophthalmic branch of trigeminal nerve (V), abducens nerve (VI)
With maxillary bone	Inferior orbital fissure	Maxillary branch of trigeminal nerve (V)
Occipital	Foramen magnum Hypoglossal canal	Medulla oblongata and accessory nerve (XI) Hypoglossal nerve (XII)
Temporal	Carotid canal External auditory meatus Internal auditory canal Stylomastoid foramen and facial nerve canal	Internal carotid artery Air in canal conducts sound to tympanic membrane Vestibulocochlear nerve (VIII) and facial nerve (VII) Facial nerve (VII)
With occipital bone	Jugular foramen	Internal jugular vein, glossopharyngeal nerve (IX), vagus nerve (X), and accessory nerve (XI)
With sphenoid and occipital bones	Foramen lacerum	Fibrocartilage, internal carotid artery as it leaves carotid canal to enter cranium, nerve of pterygoid canal, and a meningeal branch from the ascending pharyngeal artery
Maxillary	Infraorbital foramen	Infraorbital nerve and maxillary branch of trigeminal nerve (V)
Lacrimal with maxilla	Lacrimal groove, nasolacrimal canal	Lacrimal sac and nasolacrimal duct
Mandible	Mental foramen	Mental artery and nerve

187

Answers

SHORT ANSWER

1. The superior orbital fissure is located between the lesser and greater wings of the sphenoid bone in a triangular opening, for the passage of the oculomotor, trochlear, abducens, and ophthalmic division of the trigeminal nerves as well as the ophthalmic veins.
2. The mastoid antrum is located on the anterosuperior portion of the mastoid process. It is an air-filled cavity that communicates with the middle ear (tympanic cavity).
3. The middle ear consists of the tympanic membrane and the three auditory ossicles (malleus, incus, and stapes).
4. The inner ear contains the vestibule and semicircular canals, which control equilibrium and balance, and the cochlea, which is responsible for hearing.
5. The squamous suture joins the squamous portion of the temporal bone to the parietal bone.
6. The anterior fontanel is termed bregma and is located at the junction of the upper parietal and frontal bones. This fontanel remains open until age 2.
7. The anterior three fourths of the hard palate is formed by the palatine process of the maxilla, and the posterior one forth is created by the horizontal portion of the palatine bones.
8. The anterior compartment is a small cavity located anterior to the lens. It contains the cornea and iris and is filled with aqueous humor, which helps maintain intraorbital pressure. The larger posterior compartment is located behind the lens and is surrounded by the retina. The posterior compartment contains vitreous humor, which helps maintain the shape of the eyeball.

IDENTIFY

1. Figure 2.19
   a. Clivus of occipital bone
   b. Sphenoid sinus
   c. Dorsum sella of sphenoid bone
   d. Squamous portion of occipital bone

2. Figure 2.33
   a. Carotid canal
   b. Jugular foramen
   c. Sphenoid sinus
   d. Ethmoid sinus
   e. External auditory meatus
   f. Mastoid air cells

3. Figure 2.23
   a. Foramen magnum
   b. Foramen spinosum
   c. Foramen ovale
   d. Condyloid process of mandible
   e. Greater wing of sphenoid bone
   f. Clivus of occipital bone

4. Figure 2.83
   a. Pterygoid process of sphenoid bone
   b. Pterygoid hamulus of sphenoid bone
   c. Temporal bone
   d. Anterior clinoid process of sphenoid bone
   e. Sphenoid sinus
   f. Ramus of mandible

5. Figure 2.15
   a. Cribriform plate of ethmoid bone
   b. Perpendicular plate of ethmoid bone
   c. Ethmoid sinuses
   d. Anterior clinoid process of sphenoid bone

6. Figure 2.106
   a. Zygoma
   b. Ethmoid bulla
   c. Infundibulum
   d. Middle nasal meatus
   e. Uncinate process of ethmoid bone
   f. Orbital plate of frontal bone

7. Figure 2.75
   a. Palatine process of maxilla
   b. Horizontal portion of palatine bone
   c. Pterygoid process of sphenoid bone

8. Figure 2.121
   a. Optic nerve
   b. Superior rectus muscle
   c. Inferior rectus muscle

9. Figure 2.116
   a. Lens
   b. Posterior chamber
   c. Optic canal
   d. Optic nerve
   e. Medial rectus muscle

10. Figure 2.95
    a. Condyloid process of mandible
    b. Maxillary sinus
    c. Nasal septum
    d. Medial pterygoid muscle
    e. Lateral pterygoid muscle

11. Figure 2.28
    a. Hypoglossal canal
    b. Atlantooccipital joint
    c. Jugular fossa
    d. Occipital condyle

12. Figure 2.31
    a. Sphenoid sinus
    b. Dorsum sella of sphenoid bone
    c. Sella turcica of sphenoid bone
    d. External occipital protuberance

188

Answers

Copyright © 2013 by Mosby, an imprint of Elsevier Inc. All rights reserved.

13. Figure 2.40
    a. Foramen lacerum
    b. Foramen spinosum
    c. Clivus of occipital bone
    d. Jugular foramen

14. Figure 2.94
    a. Condyloid process of mandible
    b. Lateral pterygoid muscle
    c. Medial pterygoid muscle
    d. Masseter muscle

15. Figure 2.112
    a. Optic canal
    b. Superior orbital fissure
    c. Foramen rotundum
    d. Greater wing of sphenoid bone

16. Figure 2.109
    a. Optic strut
    b. Optic canal
    c. Infraorbital foramen
    d. Nasal bone

17. Figure 2.71
    a. Zygomatic arch
    b. Coronoid process of mandible
    c. Mental foramen
    d. Zygoma

18. Figure 2.65
    a. Coronal suture
    b. Squamous suture
    c. Occipitomastoid suture
    d. Lambdoidal suture

19. Figure 2.64
    a. Sagittal suture
    b. Frontal (metopic) suture
    c. Anterior fontanel (bregma)
    d. Coronal suture

20. Figure 2.62
    a. Occipital bone
    b. Internal occipital protuberance
    c. Squamous suture
    d. Temporal bone

21. Figure 2.50
    a. Lateral semicircular canal
    b. Facial nerve canal
    c. Vestibule
    d. Internal auditory canal (IAC)

22. Figure 2.51
    a. Incus
    b. Malleus
    c. Vestibule
    d. Cochlea (first turn)

23. Figure 2.52
    a. Oval window
    b. Posterior semicircular canal
    c. Cochlea
    d. Internal auditory canal (IAC)

24. Figure 2.55
    a. Mastoid antrum
    b. Stylomastoid foramen
    c. Lateral semicircular canal
    d. Occipital condyle

25. Figure 2.56
    a. External auditory meatus (EAM)
    b. Mesotympanum
    c. Vestibule
    d. Internal auditory canal (IAC)

26. Figure 2.58
    a. Incus
    b. Malleus
    c. Facial nerve canal
    d. Cochlea

27. Figure 2.21
    a. Condyloid process of mandible
    b. Dorsum sella of sphenoid bone
    c. Posterior clinoid process of sphenoid bone

28. Figure 2.9
    a. Nasal bone
    b. Frontal sinus
    c. Crista galli of ethmoid bone
    d. Ethmoid bone
    e. Meningeal groove

29. Figure 2.69
    a. Mastoid process of temporal bone
    b. Horizontal portion of palatine bone
    c. Palatine process of maxilla
    d. Zygoma

30. Figure 2.7
    a. Petrous portion of temporal bone
    b. Foramen magnum
    c. Cribriform plate of ethmoid bone
    d. Orbital plate of frontal bone

MULTIPLE CHOICE

1. b	6. b
2. a	7. a
3. a	8. c
4. c	9. b
5. d	10. c

189

CASE STUDIES

Case Study 1

1. The cranial bones typically fractured in a basilar skull fracture most often include the temporal and occipital bones, but may also involve the sphenoid and ethmoid bones.
2. Basilar skull fractures may cause tears of the meninges allowing cerebrospinal fluid (CSF) to leak through the ear structures (otorrhea) or into the nose (rhinorrhea).

Case Study 2

1. Cholesteatomas are epidermoid cysts of the middle ear.
2. The ossicles of the middle ear are the malleus, incus, and stapes
3. Cholesteatomas can be acquired or congenital but usually occur due to poor Eustachian tube function as well as infection in the middle ear.

CHAPTER 3: BRAIN

MULTIPLE CHOICE

1. b	11. b
2. c	12. a
3. c	13. c
4. d	14. b
5. d	15. a
6. a	16. c
7. a	17. a
8. d	18. c
9. d	19. b
10. d	20. d

FILL IN THE BLANKS

1. Pyramids
2. Hippocampus
3. Cerebrum, cerebellum
4. Blood pressure, heart rate, respiratory rhythm
5. Substantia nigra
6. Motor functions
7. Cerebellar peduncles
8. Temporal
9. Lateral
10. Limbic
11. Fornix
12. Arachnoid
13. Cerebral aqueduct
14. Corpus callosum
15. Caudate nucleus, lentiform nucleus, claustrum

SHORT ANSWER

1. The subarachnoid cisterns are widened areas of the subarachnoid space. These cisterns, as well as the entire subarachnoid space, are filled with cerebrospinal fluid.
2. Cerebrospinal fluid is produced by the choroid plexus, located within the ventricles. It is reabsorbed into the dural sinuses by way of the arachnoid villi.
3. The capillaries within the brain have a unique quality: they do not allow the movement of certain molecules from their vascular compartment into surrounding brain tissue. It is this impermeability of the brain capillaries that creates the blood-brain barrier.
4. The anterior communicating, posterior communicating, posterior cerebral, anterior cerebral, and internal carotid arteries form the circle of Willis.
5. Cranial nerve V (trigeminal nerve) has three branches: ophthalmic, maxillary, and mandibular.
6. Broca's area lies unilaterally on the inferior surface of the frontal lobe that is dominant for language, typically in the left frontal gyrus. This area is involved in the coordination or programming of motor movements for the production of speech sounds.
7. The frontal lobe mediates a wide variety of functions such as reasoning, judgment, emotional response, planning and execution of complex actions, and control of voluntary muscle movement. The frontal lobe is also involved with the production of speech and contains the motor speech center.
8. Heschl's gyrus is located on the superior temporal gyrus of the temporal lobe and is the primary auditory area that receives the major auditory sensory information from the cochlea.
9. The pineal gland secretes the hormone melatonin, which aids in the regulation of day/night cycles and reproductive functions.
10. Posterior inferior cerebellar artery (PICA), anterior inferior cerebellar artery (AICA), superior cerebellar artery (SCA), and posterior cerebral artery (PCA)

FILL IN THE TABLE

Cranial Nerves (see Table 3.5)

Cranial Nerves	Type	Foramen	Function
Optic (II)	Sensory	Optic foramen	Vision
Oculomotor (III)	Motor	Superior orbital fissure	Eye movement
Trochlear (IV)	Motor	Superior orbital fissure	Eye movement

Trigeminal (V)	Mixed	Meckel's cave	Multiple
Ophthalmic (V₁)	Sensory	Superior orbital fissure	Orbital structures, nasal cavity, forehead
Maxillary (V₂)	Sensory	Foramen rotundum	Cheek, upper jaw, maxillary sinuses
Mandibular (V₃)	Mixed	Foramen ovale	Lower gums, muscles of mastication, tongue
Facial (VII)	Mixed	Internal auditory canal, facial canal, stylomastoid foramen	Facial muscles, anterior two thirds of tongue
Vestibulocochlear (VIII)	Sensory	Internal auditory canal	Hearing, equilibrium
Vagus (X)	Mixed	Jugular foramen	Pharynx, larynx, thoracic and abdominal viscera
Hypoglossal (XII)	Motor	Hypoglossal canal	Tongue muscles

Internal Carotid Artery Branches (see Table 3.2)

Artery	Region Supplied
Ophthalmic artery	Globe, orbit, frontal scalp, frontal and ethmoid sinuses
Anterior cerebral artery (ACA)	Anterior frontal lobe and medial aspect of parietal lobe, head of caudate nucleus, anterior limb of the internal capsule, and anterior globus pallidus
Middle cerebral artery (MCA)	Lateral surface of the cerebrum, insula, anterior, and lateral aspects of temporal lobe, nearly all the basal ganglia and posterior and anterior internal capsules

Vertebral and Basilar Artery Branches (see Table 3.4)

Artery	Region Supplied
Posterior inferior cerebellar (PICA)	Inferior cerebellum
Anterior inferior cerebellar (AICA)	Anterior and inferior cerebellum
Pontine vessels	Pons
Superior cerebellar (SCA)	Superior cerebellum and portions of midbrain and pons
Posterior cerebral artery (PCA)	Occipital and temporal lobes

IDENTIFY

1. Figure 3.70
   a. Anterior median fissure
   b. Olive
   c. Inferior cerebellar peduncle
   d. Fourth ventricle

2. Figure 3.146
   a. Cochlea
   b. Fourth ventricle
   c. Cranial nerve VIII
   d. Cranial nerve VII

3. Figure 3.64
   a. Cerebral peduncle
   b. Red nucleus
   c. Ambient cistern with posterior cerebral artery
   d. Middle cerebral artery

4. Figure 3.65
   a. Lateral fissure
   b. Insula
   c. Quadrigeminal cistern
   d. Third ventricle
   e. Tectum (colliculi)
   f. Cerebellum

5. Figure 3.36
   a. Insula
   b. Frontal lobe
   c. Posterior commissure
   d. Lateral ventricle (occipital horn)
   e. Thalamus

6. Figure 3.31
   a. Septum pellucidum
   b. Third ventricle
   c. Thalamus
   d. Genu of corpus callosum
   e. Splenium of corpus callosum
   f. Lateral ventricle

7. Figure 3.121
   a. Calcified choroid plexus in occipital horn of lateral ventricle
   b. Great cerebral vein
   c. Internal cerebral vein
   d. Thalamostriate vein
   e. Straight sinus

8. Figure 3.16
   a. Fourth ventricle
   b. Tentorium cerebelli
   c. Medulla oblongata
   d. Corpus callosum
   e. Occipital horn of lateral ventricle with choroid plexus

9. Figure 3.72
   a. Olive
   b. Colliculi
   c. Cerebral aqueduct
   d. Cerebral peduncle
   e. Pineal gland
   f. Fornix

10. Figure 3.28
    a. Insula
    b. Parahippocampal gyrus (hippocampus)
    c. Pons
    d. Third ventricle
    e. Thalamus

11. Figure 3.47
    a. Infundibulum
    b. Head of caudate nucleus
    c. Optic chiasm
    d. Pituitary gland

12. Figure 3.30
    a. Rostrum of corpus callosum
    b. Splenium of corpus callosum
    c. Tentorium cerebelli
    d. Pineal gland
    e. Genu of corpus callosum
    f. Cerebral peduncle of midbrain

13. Figure 3.46
    a. Mamillary bodies
    b. Cerebellar tonsil
    c. Colliculi
    d. Fourth ventricle
    e. Optic nerve

14. Figure 3.98
    a. Anterior cerebral artery
    b. Middle cerebral artery
    c. Basilar artery
    d. Anterior communicating artery

15. Figure 3.96
    a. Posterior cerebral artery
    b. Basilar artery
    c. Vertebral artery
    d. Superior cerebellar artery

16. Figure 3.105
    a. Superior sagittal sinus
    b. Great cerebral vein
    c. Sigmoid sinus
    d. Straight sinus

17. Figure 3.15
    a. Corpus callosum (body)
    b. Third ventricle
    c. Temporal horn of lateral ventricle
    d. Lentiform nucleus

192

18. Figure 3.87
    a. Anterior communicating artery
    b. Anterior cerebral artery
    c. Middle cerebral artery
    d. Posterior cerebral artery

19. Figure 3.10
    a. Anterior horn of right lateral ventricle
    b. Fornix
    c. Third ventricle
    d. Occipital horn of lateral ventricle with choroid plexus

20. Figure 3.12
    a. Petrous portion of temporal bone
    b. Fourth ventricle
    c. Temporal horn of right lateral ventricle
    d. Frontal lobe

21. Figure 3.21
    a. Suprasellar cistern
    b. Interpeduncular cistern
    c. Ambient cistern
    d. Quadrigeminal cistern

22. Figure 3.34
    a. Anterior commissure
    b. Third ventricle
    c. Pineal gland
    d. Occipital horn of lateral ventricle

23. Figure 3.44
    a. Internal capsule
    b. Head of caudate nucleus
    c. Lentiform nucleus
    d. Optic chiasm

24. Figure 3.48
    a. Infundibulum
    b. Pituitary gland
    c. Sphenoid sinus
    d. Meckel's cave

25. Figure 3.57
    a. Fornix
    b. Posterior commissure
    c. Pons
    d. Parahippocampal gyrus (hippocampus)

26. Figure 3.83
    a. Internal carotid artery in carotid canal
    b. Internal auditory canal
    c. Cochlea
    d. External auditory meatus

27. Figure 3.86
    a. Carotid siphon
    b. Basilar artery
    c. Posterior inferior cerebellar artery
    d. Vertebral artery

28. Figure 3.100
    a. Anterior cerebral artery
    b. Posterior cerebral artery
    c. Internal carotid artery
    d. Middle cerebral artery

29. Figure 3.126
    a. Hypothalamus
    b. Infundibulum
    c. Pituitary gland
    d. Olfactory nerve (CN I)

30. Figure 3.19
    a. Cerebellum
    b. Fourth ventricle
    c. Tentorium cerebelli
    d. Calcified choroid plexus in occipital horn of lateral ventricle

31. Figure 3.23
    a. Cerebellopontine angle (CPA) cistern
    b. Prepontine cistern
    c. Basilar artery
    d. Pons

32. Figure 3.37
    a. Lateral fissure
    b. Suprasellar cistern
    c. Head of the caudate nucleus
    d. Temporal lobe

33. Figure 3.69
    a. Pituitary gland
    b. Thalamus
    c. Midbrain
    d. Medulla oblongata
    e. Tectum (colliculi)

34. Figure 3.85
    a. Ophthalmic artery
    b. Internal carotid artery (cavernous segment C4)
    c. Internal carotid artery (cervical segment C1)
    d. Posterior cerebral artery

35. Figure 3.90
    a. Middle cerebral artery (insular M2 segment)
    b. Middle cerebral artery bifurcation
    c. Middle cerebral artery (horizontal M1 segment)
    d. Posterior communicating artery
    e. Basilar artery bifurcation

36. Figure 3.116
    a. Trochlear nerve (CN IV)
    b. Trigeminal nerve ophthalmic division (CN V)
    c. Sphenoid sinus
    d. Oculomotor nerve (CN III)

37. Figure 3.56
    a. Ethmoid sinuses
    b. Olfactory tract
    c. Frontal lobe

38. Figure 3.135
    a. Oculomotor nerve (CN III)
    b. Cerebral peduncle
    c. Cerebral aqueduct

39. Figure 3.136
    a. Trochlear nerve (CN IV)
    b. Tectum (colliculi)
    c. Vermis of cerebellum
    d. Ambient cistern

40. Figure 3.150
    a. Vagus nerve (CN X)
    b. Vertebral artery
    c. Olive
    d. Glossopharyngeal nerve (CN IX)

CASE STUDIES

Case Study 1

1. The epidural space is located between the dura mater and the cranium.
2. The subdural space is located between the dura mater and the arachnoid membrane.

Case Study 2

1. The most common cause of a SAH is due to a ruptured aneurysm.
2. Blood will be visualized in the subarachnoid space, primarily in the basal cisterns.

Case Study 3

1. An arterial venous malformation (AVM) is a congenital type of vascular malformation that consists of a tangle of dilated arteries and veins.
2. Most neurologic AVMs cause very few if any significant symptoms. Generalized seizures and headaches can be symptoms of an AVM.
3. Approximately 40% of individuals with AVMs will bleed by the age of 40 years.

CHAPTER 4: SPINE

MULTIPLE CHOICE

1. d	6. b
2. a	7. c
3. c	8. d
4. a	9. b
5. b	10. a

FILL IN THE BLANKS

1. Denticulate ligaments
2. Pedicles, spinous
3. Brachial
4. Efferent (motor)
5. T12-L1
6. Basivertebral

7. Sciatic
8. Splenius
9. Transverse foramina
10. 31

SHORT ANSWER

1. Nucleus pulposus and annulus fibrosis make up the intervertebral disk.
2. The erector spinae muscle group is the chief extensor of the vertebral column.
3. The ligamenta flava join the laminae of adjacent vertebral arches to help preserve the normal curvature of the spine.
4. The vertebral arch is formed the pedicles (2), laminae (2), spinous process (1), transverse processes (2), and superior (2) and inferior (2) articular processes.
5. The costal facets are located on the body and transverse process, which articulate with the ribs. The head of the rib articulates with the vertebral bodies at the costovertebral joints, and the tubercle of the ribs articulates with the transverse processes at the costotransverse joints.
6. The white matter comprises the external borders of the cord and is more abundant than the gray matter. The gray matter is centrally located and surrounds the central canal.
7. The cervical plexus arises from the upper four ventral rami of C1-C4 to innervate the neck, the lower part of the face and ear, the side of the scalp, and the upper thoracic area. The major motor branch of this plexus is the phrenic nerve.
8. The sciatic nerve divides into the tibial and peroneal nerves, which innervate the posterior aspect of the lower extremity.
9. The veins of the vertebral column form an extensive network of internal and external venous plexuses, named according to their corresponding location to the vertebral column. The internal venous plexuses lie within the vertebral canal in the epidural space.
10. Iliocostalis layer (lateral column), longissimus layer (intermediate column), and spinalis layer (medial column) are the three vertical columns of the erector spinae muscle groups.

TRUE/FALSE

1. True
2. True
3. False—The transversospinal group is actually the deepest layer of the spinal muscle groups.
4. True
5. False—The cervical plexus actually arises from the ventral rami of C1-C4.
6. True
7. False—The transverse ligament is sometimes called the cruciform ligament.
8. True
9. True
10. False—The central canal is continuous with the ventricles of the brain

194

IDENTIFY

1. Figure 4.10
   a. Nucleus pulposus
   b. Annulus fibrosus
   c. Superior articular process
   d. Inferior articular process
   e. Zygapophyseal joint (facet joint)

2. Figure 4.4
   a. Body
   b. Pedicle
   c. Lamina
   d. Transverse process
   e. Spinous process
   f. Vertebral foramen

3. Figure 4.71
   a. Intervertebral disk
   b. Posterior longitudinal ligament
   c. Conus medullaris
   d. Cauda equina
   e. Subarachnoid space with CSF

4. Figure 4.14
   a. Anterior arch
   b. Posterior arch
   c. Lateral mass
   d. Transverse foramen
   e. Odontoid process of C2

5. Figure 4.37
   a. Ilium
   b. Sacral foramina
   c. Lateral mass
   d. Sacroiliac joint
   e. Body of S1

6. Figure 4.45
   a. Ligamentum nuchae
   b. Spinal cord
   c. Transverse ligament
   d. Odontoid process of C2
   e. Lateral mass of C1

7. Figure 4.67
   a. Psoas muscle
   b. Transversospinal muscle group
   c. Longissimus muscle
   d. Iliocostalis muscle
   e. Ligamenta flava

8. Figure 4.79
   a. Epidural fat
   b. Dorsal root
   c. Ventral root
   d. Conus medullaris
   e. Costovertebral joint

9. Figure 4.41
   a. Tectorial membrane
   b. Supraspinous ligament
   c. Odontoid process of C2
   d. Anterior longitudinal ligament

10. Figure 4.109
    a. Brachial plexus
    b. Left subclavian artery
    c. Right vertebral artery
    d. Right subclavian vein

11. Figure 4.85
    a. Pedicle
    b. Dorsal root ganglion
    c. Superior articular process
    d. Superior vertebral notch

12. Figure 4.15
    a. Atlantooccipital joint
    b. Lateral mass of C1
    c. Atlantoaxial joint
    d. Uncinate process

13. Figure 4.18
    a. Occipital bone
    b. Odontoid process of C2
    c. Anterior arch of C1
    d. Spinous process of C3

14. Figure 4.25
    a. Posterior thecal sac
    b. Spinal cord
    c. CSF in subarachnoid space
    d. Anterior arch of C1

15. Figure 4.42
    a. Tectorial membrane
    b. Posterior atlantooccipital membrane
    c. Transverse band of cruciform ligament
    d. Anterior longitudinal ligament

16. Figure 4.20
    a. Transverse foramen of C1
    b. Lateral mass of C1
    c. Transverse process of C3
    d. Body of C3

17. Figure 4.80
    a. Cauda equina
    b. Epidural fat
    c. Multifidus muscle
    d. Intervertebral disk (nucleus pulposus)

18. Figure 4.105
    a. Spinal cord
    b. Nerve rootlets
    c. Intervertebral foramen

195

19. Figure 4.114
    a. Internal jugular vein
    b. Subclavian vein
    c. Subclavian artery
    d. Brachial plexus

20. Figure 4.29
    a. Spinal cord
    b. Pedicle
    c. Rib
    d. Conus medullaris

21. Figure 4.30
    a. Sacral foramina
    b. Sacral promontory
    c. Coccyx

22. Figure 4.49
    a. Intervertebral disk (nucleus pulposus)
    b. Cauda equina
    c. Ligamenta flava
    d. Interspinous ligament

23. Figure 4.60
    a. Iliocostalis muscle
    b. Rotatores muscle
    c. Longissimus muscle
    d. Trapezius muscle

24. Figure 4.57
    a. Multifidus muscle
    b. Lamina
    c. Semispinalis capitis muscle
    d. Splenius capitis muscle
    e. Trapezius muscle

25. Figure 4.77
    a. Pedicle
    b. Cauda equina
    c. Conus medullaris

26. Figure 4.113
    a. Sternocleidomastoid (SCM) muscle
    b. Middle scalene muscle
    c. Brachial plexus
    d. T1

27. Figure 4.120
    a. Sacral plexus
    b. Sacroiliac joint
    c. Sacrum

28. Figure 4.131
    a. Lumbar (segmental) artery
    b. Intercostal (segmental) artery
    c. Aorta

29. Figure 4.136
    a. Basivertebral vein
    b. Thecal sac
    c. Cauda equina
    d. Psoas muscle

30. Figure 4.63
    a. Multifidus muscle
    b. Spinous process
    c. Iliocostalis thoracis muscle

CASE STUDIES

Case Study 1

1. C1 (atlas) is a ringlike structure that consists of an anterior arch, posterior arch, and two large lateral masses. C1 supports the head and articulates with the occipital condyles at the atlantooccipital joint.
2. C1 articulates with C2 (axis) at the atlantoaxial articulation. The odontoid process of C2 projects upward into the anterior ring of the atlas to act as a pivot for rotational movement of the atlas.
3. Lateral displacement of the lateral masses of C1 due to a Jefferson fracture can cause bilateral vertebral artery occlusions or transections.

Case Study 2

1. The intervertebral disks consist of a central mass of soft semigelatinous material called the nucleus pulposus and a firm outer portion termed the annulus fibrosus. The functions of these disks are to absorb shock and provide support between the vertebrae.
2. An intervertebral disk herniation is any displacement of disk material beyond the limits of the intervertebral disk space.

CHAPTER 5: NECK

MATCHING

1. a	6. c
2. b	7. f
3. e	8. d
4. g	9. i
5. h	

MULTIPLE CHOICE

1. b	6. b
2. d	7. b
3. c	8. a
4. c	9. d
5. d	10. a

FILL IN THE BLANKS

1. Piriform sinus
2. Thyroid cartilage
3. C3, C4
4. Quiet
5. Vestibular folds
6. Cricoid
7. Pharyngeal tonsils
8. Laryngeal ventricle
9. Esophageal hiatus
10. Fascial planes

FILL IN THE TABLES

Arteries of the Neck (see Table 5.4)	Origin	Branches

Common carotid artery
  Left common carotid
  Right common carotid
	
	Aortic arch
	Right brachiocephalic artery
		Internal and external carotid arteries

Internal carotid artery	Common carotid artery	Ophthalmic, anterior, and middle cerebral arteries
External carotid artery	Common carotid artery	Superior thyroid, lingual, facial, occipital, posterior auricular, and ascending pharyngeal arteries
Vertebral arteries (unite to form basilar artery)	Subclavian artery	Posterior inferior cerebellar artery

Veins of the Neck (see Table 5.5)	Termination	Tributaries
Internal jugular vein	Subclavian vein	Inferior petrosal sinus, facial, lingual, pharyngeal, superior and middle thyroid, and occasionally the occipital veins
External jugular vein	Subclavian vein	Retromandibular, anterior jugular, temporal, maxillary veins, and occasionally the occipital vein
Vertebral veins	Brachiocephalic vein	Internal and external vertebral venous plexuses and deep cervical veins

TRUE/FALSE

1. False—The cricoid cartilage is a single complete ring that forms the base of the larynx.
2. True
3. False—The false vocal cords (vestibular folds) are situated superior to the true vocal cords.
4. True
5. False—The carotid sheath encloses the common and internal carotid arteries, internal jugular vein, associated lymph nodes, and vagus nerve.
6. True
7. True
8. False—The submandibular duct is also referred to as Wharton's duct.
9. False—Approximately 10 to 20 sublingual ducts open in the floor of the mouth.
10. True

SHORT ANSWER

1. The oropharynx is a posterior extension of the oral cavity and extends from the soft palate to the level of the hyoid bone.

2. Arytenoids, corniculate, and cuneiform are the three paired cartilages of the larynx.
3. The internal jugular veins drain blood from the brain and superficial parts of the face and neck.
4. The right common carotid artery arises from the brachiocephalic artery.
5. The parotid glands are situated in front of the auricle, wedged between the ramus of the mandible and the sternocleidomastoid muscle, and extend inferiorly from the level of the external auditory meatus to the angle of the mandible.
6. The parotid gland contains fatty tissue and intraglandular lymph nodes.
7. The thyroid gland excretes the hormones, thyroxine (T4) and triiodothyronine (T3).

IDENTIFY

1. Figure 5.4
   a. Valleculae
   b. Epiglottis
   c. Cricoid cartilage
   d. Oropharynx
   e. Nasopharynx

2. Figure 5.5
   a. Tongue
   b. Pharyngeal tonsil
   c. Hyoid bone
   d. Thyroid gland

3. Figure 5.11
   a. Epiglottis
   b. Internal jugular vein
   c. Vallecula
   d. Hyoid bone
   e. Sternocleidomastoid muscle

4. Figure 5.25
   a. Epiglottis
   b. Submandibular gland
   c. Internal jugular vein
   d. Genioglossus muscle

5. Figure 5.65
   a. Hyoid bone
   b. Internal jugular vein
   c. Common carotid artery
   d. Platysma muscle

6. Figure 5.67
   a. Thyroid cartilage
   b. Vertebral artery
   c. Cricoid cartilage
   d. Internal jugular vein

7. Figure 5.48
   a. Thyroid gland
   b. Internal jugular vein
   c. External jugular vein
   d. Esophagus

8. Figure 5.13
   a. Masseter muscle
   b. Mandible
   c. Submandibular gland
   d. Aryepiglottic fold
   e. Cricoid cartilage

9. Figure 5.15
   a. Internal jugular vein
   b. Common carotid artery
   c. Epiglottis
   d. Trachea
   e. Thyroid gland

10. Figure 5.14
    a. Palatine tonsil
    b. Piriform sinus
    c. Arytenoid cartilage
    d. Cricoid cartilage

11. Figure 5.38
    a. Vertebral artery
    b. Brachial plexus
    c. Sternocleidomastoid muscle
    d. Parotid gland

12. Figure 5.36
    a. Parotid gland
    b. Retromandibular vein
    c. Medial pterygoid muscle
    d. Soft palate

13. Figure 5.43
    a. Mylohyoid muscle
    b. Genioglossus muscle
    c. Sublingual gland
    d. Internal carotid artery
    e. External carotid artery

14. Figure 5.10
    a. Sternocleidomastoid muscle
    b. Valleculae
    c. Hyoid bone
    d. Splenius capitis muscle

15. Figure 5.64
    a. Submandibular gland
    b. Sternohyoid muscle
    c. Inferior constrictor muscle
    d. Longus colli muscle
    e. Common carotid artery

16. Figure 5.24
    a. Internal jugular vein
    b. Vertebral artery
    c. Valleculae
    d. Geniohyoid muscle

17. Figure 5.26
    a. Glottis
    b. Cricoid cartilage
    c. Arytenoid cartilage
    d. Platysma muscle

18. Figure 5.28
    a. Thyroid gland
    b. Esophagus
    c. Cricoid cartilage
    d. Thyrohyoid muscle

19. Figure 5.16
    a. Piriform sinus
    b. Aryepiglottic fold
    c. Inferior constrictor muscle
    d. Sternohyoid muscle
    e. Trapezius muscle
    f. Levator scapulae muscle

198

Answers

20. Figure 5.68
    a. Sternocleidomastoid muscle
    b. Thyroid gland
    c. Trachea
    d. Esophagus
    e. Longus capitis muscle
    f. Common carotid artery

21. Figure 5.85
    a. Subclavian artery
    b. External carotid artery
    c. Brachiocephalic artery
    d. Internal carotid artery
    e. Common carotid artery
    f. Vertebral artery

22. Figure 5.84
    a. Vertebral artery
    b. Basilar artery
    c. Aortic arch
    d. External carotid artery
    e. Subclavian artery

23. Figure 5.83
    a. Common carotid artery
    b. External carotid artery
    c. Carotid artery bifurcation
    d. Internal carotid artery

CASE STUDIES

Case Study 1

1. There are nine cartilages that form the skeleton of the larynx: one epiglottis, one thyroid, one cricoid, two arytenoids, two corniculate, and two cuneiform.
2. The true and false vocal cords are important structures located in the larynx.

Case Study 2

1. The common carotid arteries bifurcate at the level of the thyroid cartilage (C3-C4).
2. The dilatation at the origin of the internal carotid artery is called the carotid sinus. It contains baroreceptors which react to changes in arterial blood pressure.

CHAPTER 6: THORAX

MULTIPLE CHOICE

1. d	6. d
2. b	7. c
3. a	8. b
4. b	9. d
5. d	10. b

FILL IN THE BLANKS

1. Pericardium
2. Myocardium
3. Hilum
4. Pulmonary veins
5. Subepicardial fat

6. Cardiophrenic sulcus
7. Right coronary artery
8. Lymph nodes
9. Thoracic inlet
10. Costophrenic sulcus
11. Costodiaphragmatic
12. Tertiary or segmental bronchi
13. Crura
14. Mammary
15. Thymosin

MATCHING

1. f	7. k
2. e	8. h
3. g	9. d
4. b	10. c
5. l	11. i
6. a	12. j

HEART MAP

8	Aortic semilunar valve
15	Pulmonary semilunar valve
7	Bicuspid valve
13	Tricuspid valve
17	Aorta
2	Left common carotid artery
5	Pulmonary veins
4	Pulmonary arteries
12	Inferior vena cava
16	Superior vena cava
1	Brachiocephalic artery
10	Interventricular septum
14	Right atrium
6	Left atrium
11	Right ventricle
9	Left ventricle
3	Left subclavian artery

SHORT ANSWER

1. Any six of the following are located within the mediastinum: thymus gland, trachea, esophagus, lymph nodes, thoracic duct, heart and great vessels, and various nerves.
2. The thymus gland is considered the primary lymphatic organ responsible for the development of cellular immunity. T-lymphocytes reach the thymus as stem cells. They are stored in the thymus while they undergo T-cell differentiation and maturation.
3. The thoracic duct drains all the lymph fluid from tissues below the diaphragm and from the left side of the body above the diaphragm.
4. Deoxygenated blood is brought to the right atrium from the inferior and superior vena cavae. The right

atrium contracts, forcing blood through the tricuspid valve into the right ventricle. The right ventricle pumps blood through the pulmonary semilunar valve to the pulmonary arteries, which enter the lungs. Oxygenated blood returns to the heart via the pulmonary veins, which enter the left atrium. The left atrium forces blood through the bicuspid valve into the left ventricle, where it is then pumped through the aortic semilunar valve to the aorta.

5. Use the horizontal long axis (HLA) image to prescribe the oblique plane through the right and left ventricles, oriented perpendicular to the interventricular septum.
6. The brachiocephalic trunk, left common carotid artery, and left subclavian artery are the three main branches of the aortic arch.
7. Left and right brachiocephalic veins are the tributaries of the superior vena cava.
8. The coronary sinus is a wide venous channel situated in the posterior part of the coronary sulcus and is the main vein of the heart.
9. The azygos venous system provides collateral circulation between the inferior and superior venae cavae.

10. The subcutaneous layer, mammary layer, and retromammary layer are the three layers of breast tissue.

TRUE/FALSE

1. False—The oblique fissure separates the inferior lobe of the right lung from the middle and superior lobes.
2. True
3. False—The parietal pleura is the outer layer of the pleura.
4. False—At approximately the level of T4-T5
5. True
6. True
7. False—It is located at the juncture of the right ventricle and pulmonary trunk.
8. True
9. True
10. True

FILL IN THE TABLE

Muscles of the Anterior and Lateral Walls of the Thorax (see Table 6.6)

Muscle	Origin	Insertion	Action
Pectoralis major	Clavicular head—medial half of clavicle. Sternal head—lateral manubrium and sternum, six upper costal cartilages	Bicipital groove of humerus and deltoid tuberosity	Flexes and adducts and medially rotates arm and accessory for inspiration
Pectoralis minor	Anterior surface of ribs 3-5	Coracoid process of the scapula	Elevates ribs of scapula, protracts scapula, and assists serratus anterior
Subclavius	First rib and cartilage	Inferior surface of the clavicle	Depresses the shoulder and assists pectoralis in inspiration
Serratus anterior	Angles of superior 8-9 ribs	Medial border of scapula	Laterally rotates and protracts scapula.

IDENTIFY

1. Figure 6.12
   a. Thoracic aorta
   b. Left oblique fissure
   c. Right oblique fissure
   d. Right cardiophrenic sulcus

2. Figure 6.18
   a. Esophagus
   b. Left mainstem bronchus
   c. Left pulmonary artery
   d. Left apical segmental bronchus

3. Figure 6.38
   a. Ascending aorta
   b. Left ventricle
   c. Right atrium
   d. Pulmonary trunk

4. Figure 6.49
   a. Right atrium
   b. Right pulmonary vein
   c. Left ventricle
   d. Right ventricle

200

5. Figure 6.93
   a. Left atrium
   b. Right atrium
   c. Right pulmonary artery
   d. Ascending aorta

6. Figure 6.99
   a. Left brachiocephalic vein
   b. Left subclavian artery
   c. Right brachiocephalic vein
   d. Brachiocephalic trunk

7. Figure 6.144
   a. Superior vena cava
   b. Azygos vein
   c. Hemiazygos vein
   d. Pulmonary trunk
   e. Descending aorta

8. Figure 6.159
   a. Pectoralis major muscle
   b. Subcutaneous fat
   c. Glandular tissue
   d. Retromammary layer

9. Figure 6.47
   a. Ascending aorta
   b. Pulmonary trunk
   c. Left atrium
   d. Descending aorta

10. Figure 6.52
    a. Interventricular septum
    b. Left atrioventricular (AV) valve
    c. Left atrium
    d. Right ventricle

11. Figure 6.80
    a. Aortic arch
    b. Left atrium
    c. Right pulmonary artery
    d. Left pulmonary artery

12. Figure 6.91
    a. Left pulmonary artery
    b. Left ventricle
    c. Right ventricle
    d. Pulmonary semilunar valve

13. Figure 6.101
    a. Brachiocephalic trunk
    b. Left common carotid artery
    c. Left subclavian artery
    d. Aortic arch

14. Figure 6.104
    a. Right coronary artery
    b. Left anterior descending artery
    c. Left circumflex artery
    d. Superior vena cava

15. Figure 6.106
    a. Left ventricle
    b. Right ventricle
    c. Right coronary artery
    d. Pulmonary trunk

16. Figure 6.109
    a. Left anterior descending artery
    b. Obtuse marginal branch of left coronary artery
    c. Diagonal branch of left anterior descending coronary artery
    d. Left circumflex artery

17. Figure 6.24
    a. Segmental bronchus
    b. Segmental pulmonary vein
    c. Descending aorta

18. Figure 6.29
    a. Brachiocephalic artery
    b. Esophagus
    c. Trachea
    d. Right brachiocephalic vein

19. Figure 6.122
    a. Left superior pulmonary vein
    b. Bicuspid valve
    c. Papillary muscle
    d. Left atrium

20. Figure 6.152
    a. Right brachiocephalic vein
    b. Pulmonary trunk
    c. Left ventricle
    d. Inferior vena cava

21. Figure 6.50
    a. Right ventricle
    b. Left ventricle
    c. Hemiazygos vein
    d. Coronary sinus

22. Figure 6.61
    a. Left mainstem bronchus
    b. Left atrium
    c. Right pulmonary artery
    d. Ascending aorta

23. Figure 6.76
    a. Superior vena cava (SVC)
    b. Right ascending pulmonary artery
    c. Left descending pulmonary artery
    d. Left inferior pulmonary vein

201

24. Figure 6.79
    a. Left pulmonary artery
    b. Right ascending pulmonary artery
    c. Right pulmonary artery
    d. Left atrium

25. Figure 6.97
    a. Left common carotid artery
    b. Left subclavian artery
    c. Right subclavian artery
    d. Right common carotid artery

26. Figure 6.111
    a. Left atrium
    b. Left circumflex artery
    c. Pulmonary trunk
    d. Left anterior descending artery (LAD)

27. Figure 6.113
    a. Left anterior descending artery (LAD)
    b. Bicuspid valve
    c. Right coronary artery
    d. Left atrium

28. Figure 6.119
    a. Great cardiac vein
    b. Left atrium
    c. Coronary sinus
    d. Left posterior ventricular vein

29. Figure 6.136
    a. Left mainstem bronchus
    b. Left pulmonary vein
    c. Left atrium
    d. Pulmonary trunk
    e. Right ventricle

CASE STUDIES

Case Study 1
1. The superior thoracic aperture is formed by the first thoracic vertebra, first pair of ribs and their costal cartilages, and manubrium.
2. The superior thoracic aperture allows for the passage of nerves, vessels, and viscera from the neck into the thoracic cavity. These include the esophagus, trachea, carotid arteries, jugular veins, and the phrenic and vagus nerves.

Case Study 2
1. It is considered the primary lymphatic organ responsible for the development of cellular immunity. T-lymphocytes within the blood reach the thymus as stem cells, where they are stored while they undergo T-cell differentiation and maturation. The thymus gland produces a hormone, thymosin, that is responsible for the development and maturation of lymphocytes.

2. The thymus gland is a triangular-shaped bilobed gland of lymph tissue, located in the superior portion of the mediastinum just behind the manubrium.

CHAPTER 7: ABDOMEN

MULTIPLE CHOICE

1. a	9. a
2. a	10. c
3. c	11. b
4. c	12. d
5. d	13. c
6. a	14. a
7. c	15. c
8. a	

MATCHING

1. e
2. b
3. a
4. d
5. c

ASSOCIATION

1. R	7. R
2. P	8. R
3. R	9. P
4. P	10. R
5. P	11. R
6. P	

FILL IN THE BLANKS

1. Glisson's capsule
2. Bare area
3. Common hepatic duct
4. Main pancreatic duct (duct of Wirsung)
5. Portal splenic confluence
6. Red and white
7. Renal (Gerota's) fascia
8. Renal pyramids
9. Ligament of Treitz
10. Haustra

SHORT ANSWER

1. The peritoneum is divided into the parietal peritoneum, which lines the abdominal walls, and the visceral peritoneum, which covers the organs.
2. The celiac trunk divides into the left gastric, common hepatic, and splenic arteries.
3. The superior mesenteric artery arises from the aorta just below the origin of the celiac trunk and passes posterior to the neck of the pancreas as it travels inferiorly to supply blood to the proximal portion of the colon and all of the small bowel except the duodenum.

4. The mesentery is a double layer of peritoneum that encloses the intestine and attaches it to the abdominal wall.
5. The peritoneal ligaments connect an organ with another organ or the abdominal wall.
6. Gastrosplenic and lienorenal ligaments attach the spleen to the greater curvature of the stomach and the left kidney.
7. Epinephrine and norepinephrine are produced by the adrenal medulla.
8. The kidneys can be divided into five segments according to their vascular supply: apical, anterosuperior, anteroinferior, inferior, and posterior.
9. The portal vein forms posterior to the pancreas from the junction of the superior mesenteric and splenic veins.
10. Abdominal lymph nodes occur in chains along main branches of the arteries of the intestine and abdominal aorta.

IDENTIFY

1. Figure 7.5
   a. Abdominal aorta
   b. Portal vein
   c. Inferior vena cava
   d. Body of pancreas
   e. Spleen

2. Figure 7.19
   a. Bare area of liver
   b. Right subphrenic compartment
   c. Left subphrenic compartment
   d. Spleen
   e. Stomach
   f. Azygos vein

3. Figure 7.84
   a. Left kidney
   b. Pancreas
   c. Portal vein
   d. Inferior vena cava

4. Figure 7.25
   a. Anterior pararenal space
   b. Renal (Gerota's) fascia
   c. Renal pelvis of kidney
   d. Abdominal aorta
   e. Posterior pararenal space

5. Figure 7.82
   a. Head of pancreas
   b. Gallbladder
   c. Left renal vein
   d. Duodenum
   e. Superior mesenteric artery
   f. Superior mesenteric vein

6. Figure 7.95
   a. Adrenal gland
   b. Crus of diaphragm
   c. Celiac trunk
   d. Spleen

7. Figure 7.92
   a. Crus of diaphragm
   b. Adrenal gland
   c. Kidney
   d. Spleen

8. Figure 7.110
   a. Psoas muscle
   b. Inferior vena cava
   c. Ureter
   d. External oblique muscle

9. Figure 7.152
   a. Celiac trunk
   b. Splenic artery
   c. Common hepatic artery
   d. Portal vein

10. Figure 7.184
    a. Rectus abdominis muscle
    b. Linea alba
    c. Internal oblique muscle
    d. Quadratus lumborum muscle
    e. Right and left common iliac arteries

11. Figure 7.56
    a. IVC
    b. Portal vein
    c. Right hepatic vein
    d. Spleen

12. Figure 7.71
    a. Cystic duct
    b. Common hepatic duct
    c. Pancreatic duct
    d. Duodenum

13. Figure 7.75
    a. Common bile duct
    b. Superior mesenteric vein
    c. Superior mesenteric artery
    d. Inferior vena cava

14. Figure 7.98
    a. Falciform ligament
    b. Left lobe of liver
    c. Common hepatic artery
    d. Celiac trunk

15. Figure 7.111
    a. Renal pelvis
    b. Ureter
    c. Bladder
    d. Sacral ala

16. Figure 7.141
    a. Left gastric artery
    b. Splenic artery
    c. Superior mesenteric artery
    d. Common hepatic artery

17. Figure 7.156
    a. Splenic artery
    b. Common iliac artery
    c. Renal artery
    d. Common hepatic artery

18. Figure 7.26
    a. Stomach
    b. Psoas muscle
    c. Adrenal gland
    d. Renal (Gerota's) fascia

19. Figure 7.37
    a. Gastroesophageal junction
    b. Descending colon
    c. Right hepatic vein
    d. Ascending colon

20. Figure 7.79
    a. Gallbladder
    b. Superior mesenteric artery
    c. Common bile duct
    d. Duodenum

21. Figure 7.81
    a. Inferior vena cava (IVC)
    b. Duodenum
    c. Pancreas
    d. Superior mesenteric vein

22. Figure 7.89
    a. Pancreas
    b. Splenic artery
    c. Falciform ligament
    d. Inferior vena cava (IVC)

23. Figure 7.107
    a. Superior mesenteric artery
    b. Aorta
    c. Third (horizontal) portion of duodenum
    d. Ascending colon

24. Figure 7.124
    a. Superior mesenteric vein
    b. Third (horizontal) portion of duodenum
    c. Liver
    d. Transverse colon

25. Figure 7.125
    a. Pancreas
    b. Splenic vein
    c. Portal vein
    d. Cecum

26. Figure 7.168
    a. Left gastric artery
    b. Superior mesenteric artery
    c. Right renal artery
    d. Inferior mesenteric artery

CASE STUDIES

Case Study 1

1. The peritoneal cavity contains potential spaces resulting from folds of peritoneum that extend from the viscera to the abdominal wall. The supracolic compartment is located above the transverse colon.
2. The supracolic compartment contains the right and left subphrenic spaces and right and left subhepatic spaces.

Case Study 2

1. If the cancer is located in the head of the pancreas, it can compress the bile duct, resulting in obstruction to the flow of bile. This can cause an accumulation of bilirubin in the bloodstream with subsequent deposition in the skin, causing jaundice.
2. The pancreas has both an endocrine (insulin, glucagon) and exocrine (digestive enzymes) function. It delivers its endocrine hormones into the draining venous system and its enzymes into the small intestines.

CHAPTER 8: PELVIS

MULTIPLE CHOICE

1. c	9. d
2. d	10. a
3. a	11. c
4. b	12. b
5. c	13. b
6. b	14. a
7. d	15. a
8. c	

TRUE/FALSE

1. False—The internal and external iliac veins join to form the common iliac veins. The right and left common iliac veins unite to form the inferior vena cava.
2. False—Sperm are produced in the testes along with male sex hormones. The sperm are stored in the epididymis as they undergo final stages of maturation.
3. True
4. True

5. False—The psoas muscle unites with the iliacus muscle to form the iliopsoas muscle. The iliopsoas is an important muscle for flexing the leg.
6. False—The arcuate line separates the iliac fossa from the body.
7. True
8. False—The iliopsoas muscle is the most important muscle for flexing the leg.
9. True
10. True

MATCHING

1. c
2. g
3. h
4. a
5. b

6. d
7. i
8. f
9. e

FILL IN THE BLANKS

1. Broad ligament
2. Fimbriae
3. Epididymis
4. Central
5. Endometrium, myometrium, perimetrium
6. Distal
7. Rectouterine
8. Piriformis
9. Pectineal, arcuate
10. Body of the ilium

SHORT ANSWER

1. The pelvic inlet or superior aperture is measured in the anteroposterior direction from the sacral promontory to the superior margin or crest of the pubic bone. The pelvic outlet or inferior aperture is measured from the tip of the coccyx to the inferior margin of the pubic symphysis in the anteroposterior direction and between the ischial tuberosities in the horizontal direction.
2. The perineum is divided into two triangles, posterior and anterior, by joining the ischial tuberosities with an imaginary line. The posterior triangle is the anal triangle, and the anterior triangle is the urogenital triangle.
3. Gluteus maximus, medius, and minimus—these muscles function together to abduct, rotate, and extend the thigh.
4. The trigone is made up of three openings in the floor of the bladder. Two of the openings are created by the ureters, and the third opening is formed by the entrance to the urethra.
5. The fimbriae spread loosely over the surface of the ovaries. During ovulation, the fimbriae trap the ovum and sweep it into the uterine tubes.

IDENTIFY

1. Figure 8.7
   a. Sacroiliac joint
   b. Lateral mass of the sacrum
   c. Sacral foramina
   d. Ilium

2. Figure 8.29
   a. Iliopsoas muscle
   b. Acetabulum
   c. Greater trochanter of femur

3. Figure 8.3
   a. Ischial tuberosity
   b. Obturator foramen
   c. Anterior superior iliac spine
   d. Pubic symphysis
   e. Iliac fossa

4. Figure 8.27
   a. Ilium
   b. Gluteus medius muscle
   c. Gluteus maximus muscle
   d. Iliacus muscle

5. Figure 8.13
   a. Iliacus muscle
   b. Psoas muscle
   c. Ilium
   d. Obturator internus muscle
   e. Lesser trochanter of femur

6. Figure 8.44
   a. Uterus
   b. Rectum
   c. Retropubic space
   d. Rectouterine pouch
   e. Bladder

7. Figure 8.63
   a. Round ligament
   b. Uterus
   c. Rectouterine pouch
   d. Vagina
   e. Rectum

8. Figure 8.70
   a. Ovary
   b. Bladder
   c. Uterus
   d. Sacrum

9. Figure 8.95
   a. Seminal vesicles
   b. Rectum
   c. Femoral vein
   d. Bladder
   e. Acetabulum
   f. Ischial spine

10. Figure 8.96
   a. Prostate gland
   b. Corpus spongiosum
   c. Bladder
   d. Seminal vesicle
   e. Pubic symphysis
   f. Corpora cavernosum

11. Figure 8.28
   a. Rectus abdominis muscle
   b. Iliacus muscle
   c. Iliac crest
   d. Gluteus medius muscle

12. Figure 8.24
   a. Obturator internus muscle
   b. Obturator externus muscle
   c. Gluteus medius muscle
   d. Gluteus maximus muscle

13. Figure 8.34
   a. Obturator internus muscle
   b. Ischium
   c. Prostatic urethra
   d. Levator ani muscle

14. Figure 8.47
   a. Ovary
   b. Urogenital diaphragm
   c. Uterus
   d. Obturator internus muscle

15. Figure 8.90
   a. Spermatic cord
   b. Femoral artery
   c. Iliopsoas muscle
   d. Ischium

16. Figure 8.82
   a. Spermatic cord
   b. Pampiniform plexus
   c. Inguinal canal
   d. Corpus cavernosum

17. Figure 8.118
   a. Celiac trunk
   b. Inferior mesenteric artery
   c. Left internal iliac artery
   d. Common hepatic artery

18. Figure 8.6
   a. Sacroiliac joint
   b. Sacral foramina
   c. Sacral nerve
   d. Gluteus maximus muscle

19. Figure 8.19
   a. Sacroiliac joint
   b. Iliac crest
   c. Iliac fossa
   d. Ischial spine

20. Figure 8.32
   a. Spermatic cord
   b. Obturator internus muscle
   c. Levator ani muscle
   d. Coccygeus muscle

21. Figure 8.46
   a. Seminal vesicle
   b. Rectum
   c. Penile urethra
   d. Pubic symphysis

22. Figure 8.53
   a. Pubic symphysis
   b. Prostate gland
   c. Rectum
   d. Coccyx

23. Figure 8.69
   a. Ovary
   b. Bladder
   c. Suspensory ligament of ovary
   d. Endometrial layer of uterus

24. Figure 8.73
   a. Left common iliac vein
   b. Uterus
   c. Right ovary
   d. Pubis

25. Figure 8.99
   a. Anterior fibromuscular stroma
   b. Central zone of prostate
   c. Neurovascular bundle
   d. Retropubic space

26. Figure 8.104
   a. Spermatic cord
   b. Corpus cavernosum
   c. Corpus spongiosum (bulb of penis)
   d. Perineal body

27. Figure 8.125
   a. Femoral artery
   b. Femoral vein
   c. Iliopsoas muscle
   d. Sciatic nerve

CASE STUDIES

Case Study 1

1. The glandular tissue comprises two thirds of the prostate's parenchymal tissue and in sectional imaging can be divided into zonal anatomy. The four main regions are the central, peripheral, transition, and anterior fibromuscular stroma.
2. The ejaculatory ducts descend within the central zone of the gland and open into the prostatic urethra at the verumontanum.

Case Study 2

1. The inguinal canal is located just superior to the inguinal ligament, passing through the lower anterior pelvic wall.
2. The inguinal canal transmits the spermatic cord in males and the round ligament in females.

CHAPTER 9: UPPER EXTREMITY

MULTIPLE CHOICE

1. d	9. a
2. c	10. c
3. c	11. a
4. b	12. b
5. c	13. d
6. c	14. b
7. a	15. b
8. a	

TRUE/FALSE

1. False—The subscapularis tendon is the only tendon of the rotator cuff to insert on the lesser tubercle; the other three insert on the greater tubercle.
2. False—The trochlea articulates with the ulna, whereas the capitellum articulates with the radius.
3. True
4. True
5. True
6. False—The subacromial-subdeltoid bursa is the main shoulder bursa.
7. True
8. True
9. False—The radial artery begins at the level of the radial head.
10. True

FILL IN THE BLANKS

1. Coracoid process
2. Biceps brachii, long head
3. Coronoid fossa
4. Ulnar collateral
5. Brachioradialis
6. Brachial artery
7. Flexor retinaculum
8. Palmar

FILL IN THE TABLE

Muscles Connecting the Upper Extremity to the Vertebral Column (see Table 9.1)

Muscle	Origin	Insertion	Primary Actions
Trapezius	External occipital protuberance, ligamentum nuchae, spinous processes of C7-T12	Clavicle, acromion, and spine of the scapula	Stabilize, elevate, retract, and depress scapula
Levator scapula	Transverse processes of C1-C4	Superior angle and medial border of scapula	Elevates scapula
Latissimus dorsi	Spinous process of T6-T12, iliac crest, and inferior 3-4 ribs	Intertubercular groove of the humerus	Extend, medially rotate, and adduct the humerus
Rhomboid major	Ligamentum nuchae and spinous processes of C7-T1	Medial border of scapula	Retracts scapula and fixes scapula to thoracic wall
Rhomboid minor	Spinous processes of T2-T5	Medial border of scapula	Retracts scapula and fixes scapula to thoracic wall

Scapular Muscles (see Table 9.2)

Muscle	Proximal/Medial Attachment	Distal/Lateral Attachment	Primary Action
Deltoid	Clavicle, acromion, and spine of scapula	Deltoid tuberosity of humerus	Flexes and medially rotates abductor, extensor, and lateral rotator of humerus
Teres major	Inferior angle of scapula	Intertubercular groove of humerus	Adducts and medially rotates humerus
Teres minor	Axillary border of scapula	Greater tubercle of humerus	Laterally rotates humerus, stabilizes glenohumeral joint
Supraspinatus	Supraspinous fossa of scapula	Greater tubercle of humerus	Abducts humerus and stabilizes glenohumeral joint
Infraspinatus	Infraspinous fossa of scapula	Greater tubercle of humerus	Laterally rotates humerus and stabilizes glenohumeral joint
Subscapularis	Subscapular fossa of scapula	Lesser tubercle of humerus	Medially rotates humerus and stabilizes glenohumeral joint

Muscles Connecting the Upper Extremity to the Anterior and Lateral Thoracic Wall (see Table 9.3)

Muscle	Proximal/Medial Attachment	Distal/Lateral Attachment	Primary Action
Pectoralis major	Medial half of clavicle, manubrium and body of sternum, and six upper costal cartilages	Lateral lip intertubercular groove of humerus	Adducts, medially rotates, and flexes humerus
Pectoralis minor	Anterior surface of ribs 3-5	Coracoid process of the scapula	Depresses and downwardly rotates scapula, assists in scapular protraction, and stabilizes scapula
Serratus anterior	Angles of ribs 1-8 or 1-9	Medial border of scapula	Rotates, stabilizes, and protracts scapula
Subclavius	First rib and cartilage	Inferior surface of the clavicle	Stabilizes the clavicle and depresses the shoulder

Muscles of the Upper Arm (see Table 9.4)

Muscle	Proximal Attachment	Distal Attachment	Primary Action
Biceps brachii	Long head—supraglenoid tubercle of scapula Short head—coracoid process of scapula	Bicipital aponeurosis and radial tuberosity	Supinates and flexes forearm

Brachialis	Distal humerus	Ulnar tuberosity and coronoid process	Flexion of elbow joint
Coracobrachialis	Coracoid process of scapula	Middle third medial surface of humerus	Assists to flex and adduct the arm
Triceps brachii	Long head—infraglenoid tubercle of scapula Medial head—posterior surface of humerus below the radial groove Lateral head—posterior surface of humerus below greater tubercle	Proximal end of olecranon process of the ulna	Chief extensor of forearm, long head steadies head of humerus if abducted
Anconeus	Lateral epicondyle of humerus	Olecranon process of the ulna	Assists triceps brachii in extension of elbow

SHORT ANSWER

1. The TFCC, also known as the articular disk, is the major stabilizing element of the distal radioulnar joint. It originates on the medial surface of the distal radius and traverses horizontally to insert on the ulnar styloid.
2. The glenoid labrum is a fibrocartilaginous ring that deepens the articulating surface of the glenoid fossa. Three fibrous bands termed the glenohumeral ligaments contribute to the formation of the glenoid labrum.
3. The anular ligament is a ligament of the elbow. This ligament forms a partial ring around the radial head to bind it to the radial notch of the ulna.
4. Scapular spine, acromion, coracoid process, and glenoid process are the four projections of the scapula.
5. The supraglenoid tubercle and infraglenoid tubercle of the scapula serve as attachment sites for biceps brachii and triceps brachii, respectively.
6. The articular joint capsule completely encloses the shoulder joint and is quite loose to allow for extreme freedom of movement. The capsule is attached medially to the glenoid fossa of the scapula and laterally to the anatomic neck of the humerus.
7. The intercarpal ligaments support the articulations between the carpal bones.
8. The flexor retinaculum is a thick ligamentous band that stretches across the carpal tunnel to create an enclosure for the passage of tendons and the median nerve.
9. The palmar tendon group collectively flexes the fingers and wrist while the tendons of the dorsal group are considered extensors of the fingers and wrist.
10. Median ulnar, musculocutaneous, and radial nerves are the nerves that supply the muscles of the forearm and hand.

IDENTIFY

1. Figure 9.18
   a. Supraspinatus tendon
   b. Glenoid fossa
   c. Superior glenoid labrum
   d. Trapezius muscle
   e. Subscapularis muscle
   f. Acromion

2. Figure 9.15
   a. Glenoid fossa
   b. Biceps brachii tendon (long head)
   c. Coracoid process
   d. Supraspinatus muscle
   e. Deltoid muscle

3. Figure 9.10
   a. Deltoid muscle
   b. Supraspinatus muscle
   c. Infraspinatus muscle
   d. Teres minor muscle
   e. Subscapularis muscle
   f. Infraglenoid tubercle
   g. Clavicle

4. Figure 9.76
   a. Lateral epicondyle
   b. Radial head
   c. Coronoid process of ulna
   d. Olecranon process
   e. Capitellum
   f. Trochlea

5. Figure 9.91
   a. Ulnar nerve
   b. Anular ligament
   c. Radial head
   d. Radial notch
   e. Olecranon process of ulna

6. Figure 9.80
   a. Biceps brachii tendon
   b. Olecranon process
   c. Coronoid process
   d. Triceps brachii muscle
   e. Brachialis muscle

7. Figure 9.100
   a. Brachioradialis muscle
   b. Anconeus muscle
   c. Brachialis muscle
   d. Flexor digitorum profundus muscle

8. Figure 9.119
   a. Scaphoid
   b. Lunate
   c. Capitate
   d. Hamate

9. Figure 9.131
   a. Median nerve
   b. Flexor retinaculum
   c. Flexor tendons
   d. Extensor tendons
   e. Hook of hamate

10. Figure 9.9
    a. Coracoid process
    b. Supraspinous fossa
    c. Acromion process
    d. Humeral head

11. Figure 9.14
    a. Biceps brachii tendon
    b. Glenohumeral ligament
    c. Posterior labrum
    d. Scapular spine

12. Figure 9.22
    a. Coracohumeral ligament
    b. Coracoid process
    c. Coracobrachialis muscle
    d. Acromioclavicular ligament

13. Figure 9.32
    a. Transverse humeral ligament
    b. Inferior glenohumeral ligament
    c. Subscapularis muscle
    d. Posterior glenoid labrum

14. Figure 9.97
    a. Brachioradialis muscle
    b. Supinator muscle
    c. Anconeus muscle
    d. Flexor digitorum superficialis muscle

15. Figure 9.105
    a. Triceps brachii tendon
    b. Coronoid process
    c. Brachialis muscle
    d. Biceps brachii muscle

16. Figure 9.145
    a. Capitate
    b. Lunate
    c. Radius
    d. Flexor tendons

17. Figure 9.130
    a. First metacarpal
    b. Opponens pollicis muscle
    c. Flexor pollicis longus tendon
    d. Opponens digiti minimi muscle

18. Figure 9.151
    a. Dorsal interosseus muscle
    b. Palmar interosseus muscle
    c. Flexor digitorum superficialis tendon
    d. Adductor pollicis muscle

19. Figure 9.6
    a. Clavicle
    b. Supraspinatus muscle
    c. Glenoid fossa
    d. Acromion

20. Figure 9.27
    a. Coracobrachialis muscle
    b. Subscapularis muscle
    c. Teres minor muscle
    d. Subscapularis tendon

21. Figure 9. 28
    a. Coracoid process
    b. Superior glenoid labrum
    c. Inferior glenohumeral ligament
    d. Long head biceps brachii tendon

210

22. Figure 9.31
    a. Subscapularis tendon
    b. Coracobrachialis muscle
    c. Deltoid muscle
    d. Posterior labrum

23. Figure 9.66
    a. Brachialis muscle
    b. Triceps brachii muscle, lateral head
    c. Triceps brachii muscle, long head
    d. Biceps brachii muscle, short head

24. Figure 9.113
    a. Capitate
    b. First metacarpal
    c. Hook of hamate
    d. Pisiform

25. Figure 9.125
    a. Scaphoid
    b. Scapholunate ligament
    c. Hamate
    d. TFCC

26. Figure 9.133
    a. Lister tubercle
    b. Pronator quadratus muscle
    c. Median nerve
    d. Extensor carpi ulnaris tendon

CASE STUDIES

Case Study 1

1. The TFCC is a fan-shaped band of fibrous tissue that originates on the medial surface of the distal radius and traverses horizontally to insert on the ulnar styloid process.
2. The TFCC is the main stabilizing element of the distal radial ulnar joint.

Case Study 2

1. The shoulder joint capsule is strengthened by several muscles and ligaments, which include the rotator cuff muscles and the long head of the biceps brachii muscle, as well as the glenohumeral and coracohumeral ligaments.
2. There are two openings of the joint capsule. The first is to allow for the transition of the long head of the biceps brachii tendon, and the second establishes a communication between the joint and the subscapularis bursa.

CHAPTER 10: LOWER EXTREMITY

MULTIPLE CHOICE

1. c		9. b	
2. a		10. d	
3. c		11. a	
4. b		12. c	
5. b		13. c	
6. a		14. b	
7. c		15. b	
8. b			

TRUE/FALSE

1. False—The acetabular labrum creates the rim attached to the margin of the acetabulum and closely surrounds the femoral head to aid in stability of the joint. The transverse acetabular ligament is, however, a portion of the acetabular labrum that spans the acetabular notch on the inferior edge of the acetabulum.
2. True
3. False—The great saphenous vein actually ascends along the medial surface of the leg and thigh, to drain into the femoral vein near the hip joint.
4. False—The tarsal canal extends laterally between the middle and posterior facet joints to form the sinus tarsi.
5. True
6. False—The centrally located pit is termed the fovea capitis.
7. True
8. True
9. True
10. False—The oblique and arcuate popliteal ligaments help reinforce the dorsal surface of the joint capsule.

FILL IN THE BLANKS

1. Fibrous joint capsule
2. Soleal (popliteal) line
3. Anterior and posterior
4. Suprapatellar (quadriceps) bursa
5. Sustentaculum tali
6. Tarsal canal
7. Plantar aponeurosis (fascia)
8. Saphenous nerve
9. Small saphenous
10. Dorsum and sole

Muscles of the Gluteal Region (see Table 10.1)

Muscle	Proximal Insertion	Distal Insertion	Action
Gluteus maximus	Ilium, sacrum, coccyx	Gluteal tuberosity of greater trochanter	Extensor of the hip, maintains erect position of the body
Gluteus medius	Iliac crest	Greater trochanter	Abducts and medically rotates the thigh
Gluteus minimus	Gluteal surface of ilium	Greater trochanter	Abducts and medically rotates the thigh
Piriformis	Sacrum	Greater trochanter	Lateral rotation and abduction of the thigh
Obturator internus	Obturator foramen	Greater trochanter	Lateral rotation and abduction of the thigh
Obturator externus	Obturator foramen	Greater trochanter	Lateral rotation of the thigh
Superior gemellus	Ischial spine	Greater trochanter	Lateral rotation and abduction of the thigh
Inferior gemellus	Ischial tuberosity	Greater trochanter	Lateral rotation and abduction of the thigh
Quadratus femoris	Ischial tuberosity	Intertrochanteric crest	Lateral rotation of the thigh

SHORT ANSWER

1. The iliotibial band is a long, wide, band of fascia that lies over the muscles on the lateral surface of the thigh. This band is a thickening of normal fascia that surrounds the entire leg and mainly helps stabilize the knee joint but also acts in flexing and extending the knee.
2. Adduction is the primary action of the medial thigh muscles. These muscles include the gracilis, pectineus, adductor longus, adductor brevis, and adductor magnus.
3. Semitendinosus, semimembranosus, and biceps femoris are collectively known as the hamstrings.
4. Anterior, middle, and posterior facets are the three articulations of the subtalar joint.
5. The fascia of the ankle thickens in various regions of the ankle to form retinacula. The retinacula form sheaths for stabilizing tendons crossing over the joints of the ankle.

IDENTIFY

1. Figure 10.3
   a. Anterior column
   b. Posterior column
   c. Acetabular fossa
   d. Fovea capitis
   e. Acetabulum

2. Figure 10.4
   a. Tensor fasciae latae muscle
   b. Sartorius muscle
   c. Iliopsoas muscle
   d. Obturator internus muscle
   e. Superior gemellus muscle
   f. Anterior acetabular labrum
   g. Iliofemoral ligament

3. Figure 10.6
   a. Obturator internus muscle
   b. Obturator externus muscle
   c. IT band
   d. Lesser trochanter
   e. Gluteus medius muscle
   f. Gluteus minimus muscle

4. Figure 10.59
   a. Intercondylar eminence
   b. Tibial plateau
   c. Lateral meniscus
   d. Medial collateral ligament
   e. Posterior cruciate ligament

5. Figure 10.88
   a. Popliteal artery
   b. Patellar ligament
   c. Anterior cruciate ligament
   d. Posterior cruciate ligament
   e. Tibial tuberosity
   f. Gastrocnemius muscle
   g. Popliteus muscle

6. Figure 10.130
   a. Navicular
   b. Sustentaculum tali
   c. Talus
   d. Lateral cuneiform

7. Figure 10.122
   a. Cervical ligament
   b. Sinus tarsi
   c. Posterior facet of subtalar joint
   d. Extensor digitorum longus tendon
   e. Achilles tendon

8. Figure 10.127
   a. Anterior talofibular ligament
   b. Tibionavicular ligament
   c. Talus
   d. Lateral malleolus

9. Figure 10.30
   a. Sartorius muscle
   b. Iliopsoas muscle
   c. Obturator externus muscle
   d. Semimembranosus tendon

10. Figure 10.45
    a. Rectus femoris muscle
    b. Vastus medialis muscle
    c. Biceps femoris muscle (long head)
    d. Vastus lateralis muscle

11. Figure 10.49
    a. Adductor longus muscle
    b. Vastus medialis muscle
    c. Vastus lateralis muscle
    d. Rectus femoris muscle

12. Figure 10.75
    a. Posterior meniscofemoral ligament
    b. Medial meniscus
    c. Popliteus muscle
    d. Biceps femoris muscle

13. Figure 10.97
    a. Sartorius muscle
    b. Popliteal artery
    c. Gastrocnemius muscle (lateral head)
    d. Posterior cruciate ligament

14. Figure 10.107
    a. Gastrocnemius muscle (medial head)
    b. Soleus muscle
    c. Tibialis anterior muscle
    d. Popliteus muscle

15. Figure 10.109
    a. Extensor hallucis longus muscle
    b. Peroneus longus muscle
    c. Soleus muscle
    d. Flexor digitorum longus tendon

16. Figure 10.112
    a. Popliteus muscle
    b. Gastrocnemius muscle (lateral head)
    c. Soleus muscle
    d. Tibialis posterior muscle

17. Figure 10.149
    a. Cuboid
    b. Spring (plantar) ligament
    c. Flexor digitorum brevis muscle
    d. Flexor hallucis longus tendon

18. Figure 10.157
    a. Talus
    b. Calcaneus
    c. Abductor hallucis muscle
    d. Deltoid ligament

19. Figure 10.158
    a. Head of talus
    b. Cuboid
    c. Navicular
    d. Adductor digiti minimi muscle

20. Figure 10.159
    a. Navicular
    b. Cuboid
    c. Flexor digitorum brevis muscle
    d. Abductor hallucis muscle

21. Figure 10.169
    a. Left common iliac artery
    b. Right internal iliac artery
    c. Left profunda femoris artery
    d. Left popliteal artery

22. Figure 10.22
    a. Iliofemoral ligament
    b. Greater trochanter
    c. Zona orbicularis
    d. Posterior acetabular labrum

23. Figure 10.24
    a. Zona orbicularis
    b. Ligamentum teres
    c. Transverse acetabular ligament
    d. Pubofemoral ligament

24. Figure 10.45
    a. Sartorius muscle
    b. Gracilis muscle
    c. Vastus intermedius muscle
    d. Biceps femoris muscle (short head)

25. Figure 10.57
    a. Medial patellar retinaculum
    b. Medial collateral ligament
    c. Posterior cruciate ligament
    d. Biceps femoris muscle

26. Figure 10.64
    a. Popliteus muscle
    b. Soleus muscle
    c. Tibialis anterior muscle
    d. Peroneus longus muscle

27. Figure 10.67
    a. Tibialis anterior tendon
    b. Tibialis posterior tendon
    c. Flexor hallucis longus muscle
    d. Extensor digitorum longus tendon

213

28. Figure 10.87
  a. Plantaris muscle
  b. Arcuate popliteal ligament
  c. Popliteus tendon
  d. Tibialis posterior muscle

29. Figure 10.96
  a. Semitendinosus tendon
  b. Gastrocnemius muscle (medial head)
  c. IT band at Gerdy's tubercle
  d. Popliteus muscle

30. Figure 10.118c
  a. Subtalar joint
  b. Cuboid
  c. Lateral cuneiform
  d. Navicular

31. Figure 10.144
  a. Tibialis posterior tendon
  b. Flexor hallucis longus tendon
  c. Soleus muscle
  d. Posterior tibiofibular ligament
  e. Peroneus longus tendon

32. Figure 10.162
  a. Extensor hallucis tendon
  b. Plantar plate
  c. Flexor hallucis longus tendon
  d. Abductor hallucis tendon

CASE STUDIES

Case Study 1

1. The tarsal tunnel is formed by the flexor retinaculum as it stretches between the medial malleolus and the medial tubercle of the calcaneus.
2. The tibialis posterior and flexor digitorum longus tendons, flexor hallucis longus muscles, and the posterior tibial vessels and nerve pass through the tarsal tunnel.

Case Study 2

1. The lateral meniscus is most mobile because the medial meniscus is attached to the medial collateral ligament.
2. Two ligaments arise from the posterior horn of the lateral meniscus. The posterior meniscofemoral ligament (ligament of Wrisberg) passes behind the posterior cruciate ligament to attach to the medial femoral condyle. The anterior meniscofemoral ligament (ligament of Humphrey) connects the posterior horn to the medial condyle, passing in front of the posterior cruciate ligament.